THE
ATHLETE'S
PLATE

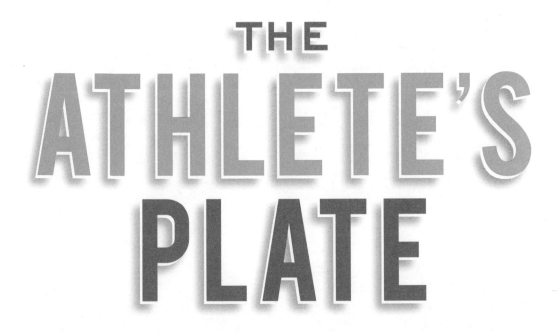

THE
ATHLETE'S
PLATE

Real Food for High Performance

ADAM KELINSON

VELO press

BOULDER, COLORADO

1830 55th Street
Boulder, Colorado 80301-2700 USA
303/440-0601 · Fax 303/444-6788 ·
E-mail velopress@competitorgroup.com

Distributed in the United States and Canada
by Ingram Publisher Services

Library of Congress Cataloging-in-Publication Data
Kelinson, Adam.
The athlete's plate: real food for high performance
/ Adam Kelinson.
    p. cm.
Includes bibliographical references and index.
ISBN 978-1-934030-46-2 (pbk. : alk. paper)
1. Athletes—Nutrition. I. Title.
TX361.A8K45   2009
613.2'024796—dc22

2009037501

For information on purchasing VeloPress books, please call 800/234-8356 or visit www.velopress.com.

This book is printed on 100 percent recycled paper (80 percent minimum recovered/recycled fiber, 30 percent post-consumer waste), elemental chlorine free, using soy-based inks.

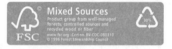

Cover design by theBookDesigners
Interior design and composition by Jane Raese
Photography by Annette Slade, www.sladephoto.com
Food styling by Jacqueline Buckner, www.food4film.com
Illustrations by Mike Reisel
Text font is Fairfield Light.

09   10   11 / 10   9   8   7   6   5   4   3   2   1

This book is dedicated to one person:

Beth

and three dogs:

Maya, Zoe, and Choden.

Without them this would not have been possible . . . and then some.

Don't give up . . . don't ever give up!
—Coach Jimmy Valvano

Contents

Recipes List

Preface

*A Lakota medicine man, Wallace Black Elk, was once asked
by a sincere young man what we could do to heal the Earth.
His reply was, "We don't have to heal the Earth; she can heal herself.
All we have to do is stop making her sick."*

—Eliot Cowan, *Plant Spirit Medicine*

I grew up in an urban environment, and the playground of my youth was filled with cars, noise, fast food, and their associated by-products. Instead of gazing at far-off peaks with a sense of adventure as I imagined climbing them, I was overshadowed by skyscrapers and wondered who already lived in their penthouses. It's funny how elevation is metaphorically related to one's awareness, because from our apartment one set of windows had a clear view of a Burger King restaurant in the street below, and the other narrowly revealed a bend in the Hudson River. It was not until many years later that the perspective from these two images truly came into focus for me.

It was high above those streets that I first realized there were more natural places to eat and play than the supermarket and sandbox. Perched within our apartment, I watched Grizzly Adams live off the land and the High Mountain Rangers blast through the backcountry on our TV. Fortunately, my parents found a way to send me off to experience some of the glory of the wide-open world during summers in the Berkshire Hills. I had the opportunity to see and explore the differences between the two places, how people choose to live, and the impact that urban living can have on the environment. But, again, I needed time to fully understand these differences.

It is also no coincidence that one of my first memories involves food. In fact, the majority of my memories relate to food in some way, even if just in remembering what I happened to be eating at the time. If food is not the theme, then a backcountry outing or athletic endeavor is. Add to this the fact that the first club of which I became a member was Greenpeace, and you can easily see the formative threads of my life. This book reflects the ways in which I have woven them together.

While other kids sought out paper routes or lawn-mowing jobs or got started in the family business, I looked for work involving food. One of my first jobs happened to be at that Burger King. Although it was not part of the job description, it was there that I saw the biggest rat of my life. I'm not an expert on rodents, but I've spent plenty of time in the forest and ridden many a New York subway, and I assure you, this critter was large! I had been lifting weights in the gym, like many athletic guys, but the size of this creature was not an inspiration to better understand what to eat in order to get big. Instead, it ensured that I had placed my last Whopper order.

In recognizing the importance of food and its connection to the land, I explored different types of diets, paying attention to how my body responded. I have been active all my life, and outdoor sports have taken me to some of the most pristine places the earth has to offer. I have climbed rock faces, ice pillars, and mountains; guided through perilous whitewater; surfed overhead waves; and tested my physical and mental strength in grueling endurance races and solo wilderness wanderings. As a result, I have touched upon the sacred connection to the earth and learned that an active lifestyle requires balance, high-quality nutrition, and a healthy planet to support it.

So it was almost déjà vu when I began to realize that a lot of athletes, like rats, had no discrimination when it came to their food choices. Thinking that all foods were the same regardless of their nutritive value, these athletes clearly had no idea how to eat to perform properly because they did not understand the connection between their bodies and their food consumption. Furthermore, they did not recognize how their food choices related to the health of the environment.

To me it seemed obvious that food, cooking, nutrition, and being active were inextricably linked in the most natural way and that the source of that link was a relationship with the earth. In my mind, how could you do one without the other?

Yet most of the sources of information on nutrition and sports ignored this link. They never made the connection that by understanding the value of your food and how it feeds you, you will begin to understand the value of where that food comes from.

The sources were deficient in other ways, too. Nutritional information should be easy to grasp, and recipes should be healthy, simple, and quick to prepare. But books on sports nutrition (I have a shelf full of them) are often so specific that they are impenetrable. And books about food for fitness are not only limited in their message but also unnecessarily complicated, with too many ingredients and too many steps. People with active lifestyles are busy, and they need accessible information on preparing nutritionally complete, quick meals that satisfy their energy needs as well as their appetites.

And let's be honest: nutrition is boring. Food is the energy source of life—it should be delicious, support an active lifestyle, and help maintain an active body. And it should be exciting! I came to understand that to get my ideas about good food and its connection to the earth across, I would need to transcend the trendy health and fitness programs that leave so many motivated individuals defeated by their inability to integrate the plans into their everyday lives.

The solution to this puzzle was simple, centuries old, and represented in the Taoist symbol of yin and yang. As Donald Reid puts it in *The Tao of Health, Sex, and Longevity*, the "way" (as *Tao* literally means) is "a trail on the journey through life which conforms to nature's own topography and time-tables, and . . . our best hope for survival is to live in harmony with the great natural forces that formed us as well as our environment."

I realized that I could use this concept to help athletes and those living active lifestyles understand that food is an inextricable link to performance, and the quality of athletic performance is determined by the quality of food consumption. Moreover, because I am a chef as well as an athlete, I could also provide recipes, cooking techniques, and information on food sources that I have used to help other athletes find success without feeling trapped by the drudgery of counting calories, constantly shopping for food, using processed supplements, and feeling isolated by a lack of comprehensible information.

Athletes can be fickle and superstitious, and they tend to like routines. It was crucial for this book, therefore, to translate the traditional lifestyle of nutritious, fresh ingredients into a system that could seamlessly fit into the busy lifestyle of an athlete while simultaneously promoting increased health and performance.

My system will integrate nutrition into your athletic lifestyle based upon a reconnection to the earth. You don't have to be an athlete to learn from it; after all, we all need food to live. Anyone can use this book to learn how to use and nourish the earth's sources to draw the benefits that nature's bounty provides.

The ideas in this book have been developing and percolating in my mind for more than 15 years. It took me that long to solidify a system that you will find sustainable for the rest of your life. My "programless program" will not leave you wondering how to incorporate it when you have finished the book. Instead, you can easily make this system a part of your daily routine, and it will make your approach to food preparation simpler and quicker than it currently is.

I ought to point out that this is not a story of regaining one's health or recovering from sickness. Instead, it is a story about how I have prevented the need to do so. Once you appreciate the power of a proper nutritional paradigm, you can regain the connection to the source of life from which it all arises. At that point, you will begin to intuitively make the best choices to support a healthier life. It's not that you have to be spiritual, but simply that you will recognize that life is filled with spirit.

Sometimes you have to get to the end of your journey in order to be able to see the whole process. And because I have already made my journey with this book, you can enter it at any chapter or page and begin to glean its lessons. It is a book of parts that make up a whole that can assist in supporting your lifestyle at any phase of your life.

Simply put, the ideas in this book have not been designed to tell you how to live but to provide you with the information, tools, and guidance to help you make the choices that best suit your own life. From there, anything is possible.

Acknowledgments

I can only hope this page serves as a reminder to all those mentioned below of my deepest gratitude, from the bottom of my heart, for being a part of this project. And that our personal interactions already made you aware of how important you are.

I would like to recognize the hero of this book, the earth, for providing us with its most precious assets.

To everyone who asked, "When are you going to write a book?" and to those who were continuously supportive in wondering, "How's it going?" thank you for the encouragement and careful thought. Here it is.

To all those who have been pioneers and, when everyone seems to be going in one direction, are—rest assured—tirelessly willing to follow another path: don't ever think your efforts were wasted; they got me here.

To everyone at VeloPress for taking a chance on an unknown author with a topic that pushes the boundaries: publisher Ted Costantino, associate publisher and editor Renee Jardine, editorial assistant Jessica Jones, project editor Connie Oehring, and marketing manager Dave Trendler. If publishing was an endurance sport, these folks would rule. And to my agent, PJ Mark, who got it. Good work!

To Barbara Dills: down and late in the fourth quarter, there is no one I would rather have on my team.

My envy and praise to all those farmers on land and sea who sustainably grow and harvest the wonderful bounty of food that inspired the recipes: the gang at the Seafood Shop, Dale and Betty, Merilee Foster, David Falkowski of Open Minded Organics, Art Ludlow of Mecox Dairy, Good Earth Farms, Quail Hill Farm, 3-Corner Field Farm, Garden of Eve Farm, and any others I regrettably forgot.

To all of my family, friends, and colleagues for their generous support: Mom, Dad, Josh, the Shekinah Cowboys, Swami Chetanananda, Lou Rotola, Karin Auwaerter, Eugene from the Beachbreak, Abu, sagg main surfers, Dani from Tropical Gardens, and Edwina von Gal. Also, everyone who took the time to be interviewed, especially Dr. John Ivy, and all those athletes willing to train and step up to the line to test themselves. You are all a constant source of inspiration.

Finally, to Maya, my daily inspiration to live in the moment with unconditional love. She has been my greatest teacher.

Keep it under the rainbow, everyone. Big loves.

—*Adam*

1

Making Nutrition a Lifestyle

Athletes are busy people. They constantly cut corners to save time and balance the demands of their sport with everything else in their lives. Inevitably, what it means to eat well and prepare fresh, whole foods is lost in the pursuit of training, racing, and recovery. Yet food is fundamental to the performance athletes seek.

When I talk with athletes about their diets, they often rattle off a few foods they eat repeatedly, often with little enthusiasm. But when I ask these same people about their bike frames, wet suits, surfboards, or shoes, they sound like salespeople at a sports gear convention. As an athlete, you have to learn to become just as passionate about the most important tool you have: your body. Your body is the engine that drives the sports equipment you adore, and that engine needs premium fuel to produce high-quality power. Indeed, because your body is the foundation of any sport, you should treat it better than any piece of gear you own. Once you become attuned to incorporating whole foods and healthy cooking into your life, great-tasting, nourishing food will become another partner in your training.

I liken this to the "zone" that athletes talk about, where practice and training blend into action and thought becomes instinct. Nutrition is no different. It is not something you should have to constantly think about as an external input; it should be something that is a seamless part of your life. Again, active lifestyles and athletes—especially endurance athletes—have particular nutritional requirements for training and racing, but the foundational concepts of this book will remain the same for the other 21 hours or so of your life that you are not working out. As such, you will not find any rules here to live by. Instead, you'll find guidelines that can fit into your own lifestyle in an effort to find your own balance.

Eating itself requires balance and can be divided into many parts: menu ideas, shopping, food storage, preparation, cooking, eating, and then cleaning up. Add to that the daily tasks of work, family, play, your personal needs, and the other bits of time that are necessary to make all of this happen, and the thought of actually cooking can become overwhelming. But it doesn't have to be. Eating can be fun and enjoyable, and cooking can be satisfying and easy, requiring little time. Cooking can, in fact, help you find balance and a connection to yourself, your family, your community, and the natural world.

Better Food, Better Performance, Better Health, Better Planet

A good nutritional program looks at more than simply what you eat. It is based on a holistic perspective that enfolds the planet and your lifestyle, and considers the quality of the food you eat, its nutritional value, and its role in supporting your life and goals.

Good nutrition also depends on good sources of food. The integrity of what you eat depends on how foods are grown, handled, and prepared. As such, nutrition is more than just being told what to eat. Its long-term success relies on a relationship that each of us fosters through our connection to ourselves and our communities, by understanding where our food comes from and how its production is attuned to the cycles and health of the earth.

For many athletes, the difficulty in crossing the bridge between what to eat and how to do it within the time constraints of an active lifestyle is the biggest challenge to success. The key is to understand that the what and the how exist in the same place. Most people look at nutrition and proper eating as an external chore outside of their daily life. But prior to the academia of nutrition, native societies lived with great health on a diet based on local foods that were seasonally available and prepared using techniques that enhanced the quantity of nutrition in each bite, and made that nutrition more available to the body. Nutrition was part of their lifestyle, and they understood where it came from and that their health and the health of the planet depended on it. Contemporary society is structured much differently, but we can still incorporate similar dietary habits and skills that will improve our health, our performance, and our daily lives.

It is hardly news that athletic performance depends on nutritional intake. There are scores of scientists, dietitians, doctors, and sports nutritionists who focus solely on the relationship between the two. But nutrition is only part of the equation. The quality of one's food, how to integrate and execute that intake into daily living, and its impact upon the earth are elements that are often ignored.

Scott Jurek, ultrarunning's most accomplished athlete, who has won the Western States 100-mile endurance run an epic seven times, puts more miles on his legs in a week than I do on my car, but he still prepares virtually all of his own food. His training philosophy is based on the idea that for his body to positively respond to the rigors of training, he needs to create lifestyle habits that promote health in all aspects of life.[1] Simply put, your lifestyle must support your nutrition, and your nutrition must support your lifestyle. This is the holistic approach that will manifest success in all areas of your performance.

You don't have to master all the components of this concept, but you do have to understand that each part is equally important to the whole. During Dave Scott's six successive Ironman® triathlon championships, he would drain cottage cheese over the sink in his hotel room to get an edge on his competitors.[2] Clearly there is some absence of culinary excellence here, but he knew how important his nutrition was to his racing and took an active part in its execution. Although most athletes want to be told what and how to eat, personal success has to include personal participation. Once you begin to learn about one area, you will see how it naturally fits with the others.

The process of getting from one side of the bridge to the other does not need to be overwhelming. The road to athletic success is paved with practice, and nutrition is just another part of that practice. In order to make nutrition part of your lifestyle, however, it helps to have reminders that assist in decision making from day to day. The following guidelines are ones that you can take with you wherever you go and can begin to use as soon as you finish reading them. They are very simple tenets to use on a daily basis when you are faced with decisions about what foods to buy, where to buy them, and how they might affect the planet. Using them will keep you living a happy, healthy, and active lifestyle through each and every permutation of your athletic career.

Keep in mind, however, that these are not steps to accomplish and check off; they are concepts to embrace. The guidelines are a structure, but within them are many choices. For example, buying local foods is something that we all can do, but which foods you buy is dependent upon your lifestyle and flavor preferences. These guidelines will reconnect you with the needs of your body as they change from sport to sport and year to year.

The Big Three

These first three steps are fundamentally important. By practicing these three you will incorporate much from the others that follow.

Buy local meat and local produce, and buy organic. Purchasing your food locally and selecting from organic foods will increase the flavor, freshness, and nutrient value of the things you eat, provide a connection point to the seasonal cycles and availability of your local foods, reduce your exposure to chemical fertilizers and pesticides, limit the impact that industrial agriculture has on the environment, support the infrastructure of your local economy, and save you precious time in your life from having to think about the best foods to buy.

In 1960, farmers made up 7 percent of the U.S. population. In 1994 that number dropped to 1.5 percent; today it is less than 1 percent in a population of 285 million. In 1935 the number of farms peaked at 6.8 million; today it is estimated as below 2 million. However, during this decline the overall population has increased along with the demand for agricultural products. According to the U.S. Environmental Protection Agency (EPA), "this increased demand has been met (and exceeded) with the aid of large-scale mechanization (the use of large, productive pieces of farm equipment), improved crop varieties, commercial fertilizers, and pesticides."[3] It is a model that has come to be known in the agricultural industry as "Get Big or Get Out"—which is exactly what has happened. As a result of this model, millions of farm families have been driven off the land, unable to compete with large-scale agribusiness. The get-big model has created a factory system of food production that has been tuned for maximum output. Yet studies have shown that yield increases "produced by fertilization, irrigation and other environmental means tend to decrease the concentrations of minerals in plants."[4] As small, localized farms have left the landscape, the families that managed them and the nutrients in the food they grew have left with them.

The rapid decline of local farms has driven our personal resources farther from our homes. The system of corporate agriculture requires the consolidation of production, and as a result the agribusiness holdings are located a great distance from the people who ultimately purchase these foods. A study in Iowa showed that conventionally grown produce travels 27 times farther on average to its point of sale than does the same produce grown locally.[5] The farther we are from the production of our food, the less we know of how it was grown; the greater the impact it has upon the environment for travel, packaging, and chemical input; the greater the opportunity it has for contamination; and the less money and jobs our local economies receive.

Buying food locally provides us with a point of access for knowing how our food is produced. You know who grows your food, where it comes from, and how it is grown. These are important factors for everyone trying to increase the health of their bodies as well as their daily performance.

"Local" does not mean that the food you eat has to come from your garden, the garden down the road, or even a farm within your community. The closer to home your food grows, the better, but "local" can encompass a valley, a watershed, a county, or a small geographic region. For instance, in New York City locally grown foods can come from a small garden in Brooklyn or from a farm 100 miles away in the Hudson Valley. What is important is to practice what Kirkpatrick Sale, in his book *Dwellers in the Land: The Bioregional Vision,* calls bioregionalism, which is the concept of getting to know the place where you live, the kinds of plants and animals that inhabit the area, the source of its waters, the soil, and its ability to sustain life within it. Having a connection to the land that supports you adds the crucial element to the sustainability equation that this symbiotic relationship requires and will help you make better decisions about how you can continue to support it.

Despite their freshness, local foods are not invariably organic, which begs the question of whether fresh, local, and conventional food is better than packaged, well-traveled organic selections. Studies have shown that the nutritive content of organically grown foods is, on average, 25 percent higher than similar foods that have been conventionally grown.[6] At the same time, freshness counts for a lot, as does the environmental impact of long-distance shipping and its required packaging. My own hierarchy is local organic first, then local conventional, and then imported organic. However, this is not written in stone. Ultimately, by purchasing as much food locally as I can, I come to know the quality of those foods and how they are grown, which are the two most critical factors regarding the food I eat. Supporting local organic farming with my purchases also encourages my community to increase the availability of real foods.

Read as few labels as possible. The idea here is simple: fewer labels means less processing. Once you are no longer shopping for fresh produce, labels are a sign that you have greatly distanced yourself from your food source and its nutrients. Labels are indicators of processing, pasteurization and/or preservatives, and, most likely, refined carbohydrates and sugars—and that is true even if the packaged food was purchased in a health food store. They are also part of a system of packaging that adds to our waste stream.

Buying packaged food is inevitable, of course. So the corollary to this rule is, always read the label before purchase. Just because something is in a package does not mean that it is safe.

Labels and packaging indicate that the food product inside is a conglomeration of multiple ingredients that have undergone extensive processing among various producers and distributors. In almost every case, each food item in a packaged product has been pooled with the same item from other sources, with each one being handled differently en route to final destination. Let's take the salmonella contamination of peanuts in February 2009 as an example. Clif Bar is a producer of sports food products, and it was one of the first such companies to use organic ingredients in its formulas. It is a brand in the sports food world that health-conscious athletes have trusted and relied on. Clif Bar sources its energy bars' many different ingredients from a number of farms and food distributors, which ship the ingredients to a central processor where the bars are made. With packaging that says "Made with Organic" on some products and the organic certification label on others, Clif Bars would appear to be a safe and healthy food source. But these labels can be confusing.

In fact, Clif Bar purchased peanuts from a company that did have organic certification for its facility. However, the peanuts in the bars were not organic. And that peanut supplier was also the one in which the salmonella contamination originated, from which nine people died and over 700 were poisoned. Reading the label may not have saved you from exposure, but it would have told you that not all of Clif Bar's ingredients were organic, the peanuts being one of them. Keep in mind that this is not an indictment of Clif Bar but an example of how mass-produced, centralized food processing has replaced our own involvement with a false sense of security that what we purchase is safe to eat.

One must also keep in mind that almost anything in a bottle or can has been pasteurized, and the majority of packaged foods as well as some meats and produce are irradiated, cooked, or heat-treated to kill off potential pathogens. These are necessary steps in the centralized food production system, which due to its size, lack of quality control, and speed of operation has created environments and conditions where harmful pathogens can thrive. Keep in mind, too, that even when foods are cooked, irradiated, or pasteurized, they can be recontaminated and sold as safe.[7] And as Rodney Leonard of the Community Nutrition Institute points out in Marion Nestle's book *Safe*

Food, irradiation is not a particularly effective weapon against contamination. As he notes, "All irradiation will do is add partially decontaminated fecal matter to the American diet, a practice that is likely to cause food poisoning cases to skyrocket when bacteria develop the survival tactics to resist irradiation. All past efforts to 'eradicate' microbial organisms . . . have succeeded only in creating new generations of super bugs, and irradiation will be no different. . . . The solution to the food safety problem is to produce safe food."[8]

Love yourself and your environment. Life is not about what you do but what you bring to it. Without caring for yourself, how can you care about others? We can all choose to eat healthier foods, but how do we make that a sustainable process? The answer that I have found is that the love we have for ourselves has to be bigger than we are. That love has to connect us with something that provides motivation and inspiration that goes beyond our own harvest. Food choices have the ability to fulfill this. We can make the decision to care for our bodies and realize the implications of caring for others as well as the environment.

Think of the future for others. Understand that we are part of nature and rely on it for our health and well-being. If we take care of it, it will take care of us.

The Supporting Cast

Embracing the preceding Big Three will lead you to incorporating the following supporting players. They are nothing more than simple guidelines to keep in mind. My intention here is not to create a list of things to avoid, give up, or agonize over. Instead, the list is intended as encouragement to help you make some better-quality choices every day. This book is aimed at simplifying your life and increasing your performance. It's about providing you with the tools and resources to help you re-create your relationship with yourself, your food, and your community. From there, you can become anything you want.

Stay away from the processed corns and their by-products. Whenever possible, avoid high-fructose corn syrup, corn solids, corn syrup, cornstarch, and its associated by-products like maltodextrin and dextrose, with the exception of that grown and produced organically. Corn, of course, has been a staple food for centuries, powering some of the world's best runners, and in its natural state it continues to be a good food source today. In the modern Western diet, however, corn has been refined and processed into almost everything you find on a shelf in a standard supermarket. Corn is used today as a sweetener for sodas, jams, fruit juices, chips, condiments, sports gels, drinks, and bars; as a flow agent and binder for pills and tablets; as a stabilizer for bread, dough, and noodles; and as a feed for beef, chicken, pork, and fish.

According to the U.S. Department of Agriculture (USDA), in 2007, Americans consumed, on average, 40.1 pounds of high-fructose corn syrup (HFCS) per person.[9] There is a continuing debate about the nega-tive health effects of HFCS as a major cause of childhood obesity and adult-onset diabetes, and many have also suggested it has been a major factor in heart disease, the increase of high blood cholesterol and triglycerides, and an increased clotting factor in red blood cells, leading to embolisms and strokes.[10]

One certainty about the overproduction of corn can be seen in its negative impact on the environment. Because corn is grown as a monoculture, where only one crop is planted over a large acreage, it requires large amounts of chemical fertilizers, pesticides, and herbicides. In addition, almost all corn used today has been genetically modified in some way to deal with the collateral issues involved with this type of growing.

Avoiding high-fructose corn syrup is not easy in processed foods, but it is easy in natural foods and when cooking at home. Honey and maple syrup are great natural sweeteners that can be found in their raw form; both contain amazing amounts of nutrients and minerals. Raw honey can generally be found locally, adding to its appeal. Other good choices include agave nectar or syrup (very low on the glycemic index) and stevia, which although not local is generally easy to find.

If you can't read it or pronounce it, don't eat it. This means the hydro's, mono's, tri's, trans', sat's, di's, phos's, pry's, -ate's, -ite's, and any combination of them. Food and eating are simple. You should not need a scientific dictionary to understand what you put in your stomach. Reducing the number of labels in your shopping cart simplifies the task of finding nutritious food. What about bottled vitamins, you ask? As you will see later in the book, if you are eating a well-balanced diet based on the principles in this chapter, you can be confident that you are getting all the nutrients your body needs without having to find them on a label. Stay as close to the tree or plant as you can. You will get all of the nutrients that you need in a much more bio-available form.

Limit your chemical exposure. Personal hygiene products and household cleaners should be biodegradable and nontoxic. When clients describe a processed food or product they use, I ask what's in it. The invariable response is, "I don't know." If most people don't even have time to eat properly, how many of us have time to research those polysyllabic words on our personal and household products? Not many.

If you were to look into them, though, you would find that they contain petroleums, solvents, alcohols, phthalates, parabens (methyl, p-propyl, isobutyl, n-butyl, benzyl), and chemical additives that are known carcinogens. These products show up in cosmetics, shampoos, sunblocks, antiperspirants, auto lubricants and waxes, paints, and other industrial uses. These everyday items might contain minute amounts within single applications, but over the course of years they add up to measurable concentrations. In particular, they have been found to be present in the blood and tissues of women who have been diagnosed with breast cancer. Household products contain bleaches, phosphates, and other substances that will either kill plants and animals directly or stimu-

late the growth of aquatic plants and algae that indirectly kill fish and overtake water bodies. Check the ingredient list on the products you use and see how many of them contain these ubiquitous chemicals.

Fortunately, there are many environmentally advanced products on the market to choose from. Many have been around for a long time and boast formulas that are just as effective as the conventional chemical products. Moreover, most are widely available; see the "Resources" chapter for more information.

Eat with the seasons. Not everyone is fortunate enough to live in an area where an abundance of fresh food is available year-round, and even those places where fresh food is available are still subject to seasonal changes. However, the seasonal guide in the "Resources" chapter will help you find and take advantage of what is available in yours. Buying locally takes the thought out of this process and helps with menu planning, since all you have to do is show up and nature's peak flavor, freshness, and nutrient content will be there, waiting for you.

Don't cook what you can eat raw; save time and nutrients. "I don't have the time to cook" is something I often hear; my response is, "Do you have time to eat?" This book is all about reducing your time in the kitchen while improving the quality of what you eat. Decreasing the time you cook food and incorporating a large percentage of raw foods in your diet will go a long way toward saving time and improving your nutrition. In addition, you will find that for many foods, long cooking reduces the flavor and nutrient quality that fresh, locally bought organic foods have to offer.

The recipes in this book will show you techniques that will help you prepare meals quickly using a combination of foods, both raw and cooked, allowing you to eat well. After all, fresh, raw food contains all of the life force and nutrients that support a living plant along with enzymes that are crucial for its digestion. When we consume a diet based entirely on cooked foods, our bodies need to supply the necessary enzymes for digestion that were destroyed by heat during cooking. Consequently, enzymes that were to be used for other purposes, such as repair and recovery of muscles, become unavailable. Our bodies do not have an endless supply of enzymes, and the perpetual and supplemental use of them in this way will eventually lead to a breakdown in the body in some fashion.[11] This is why sprouts, vegetables, and fruits that are raw and still retain their life force, along with those that are lacto-fermented, like sauerkraut, pickles, and kimchi, are so good for you.

Soak, sprout, ferment, dehydrate. Grains, seeds, legumes, and nuts are very beneficial to an athlete's diet, as are foods that have been soaked, sprouted, or fermented. The techniques are simple, but they need to be incorporated into a daily schedule. As with anything, the more you do it, the easier it becomes. If you are limited by your schedule, however, don't limit your nutrient quality and quantity as a result. If you can't fit the time for soaking, sprouting, or fermenting into your day, visit the "Resources" chapter of the book to help you figure out where you can buy foods that have already been prepared.

Include essential fatty acids and antioxidants. Essential fatty acids (EFAs) and antioxidants are important components in our daily living. EFAs are healthy fats, better known as the omegas (3 and 6), that the body cannot produce on its own. A healthy ratio of omega-6 to omega-3 is estimated to be about 4:1. However, as a result of the overconsumption of processed foods and the overuse of polyunsaturated vegetable oils and substitute fats, says Jeffery Boost, PAC, who collaborated on two studies on the levels of omega-3 in athletes' diets, 90 percent of Americans are deficient in omega-3s and have an abundance of omega-6. While omega-6 is essential, its pro-inflammatory abilities have been seen as a potential risk of heart disease when excessive amounts are present.[12] The recipes in this book will supply omegas along with antioxidants in your meals in the proper ratios, but it is important to be aware of their intake, as you are ultimately responsible for your own diet. Some of the better sources of EFAs are:

- Seeds and their oils: flax, hemp seed, coconut, and pumpkin.
- Nuts: walnuts, almonds, and cashews.
- Deep-sea fish: mackerel, bluefish, and fish oils.
- Blue-green algae: chlorella, spirulina, and leafy green vegetables are great plant-based sources.

Some reasons to incorporate EFAs into your diet are:

- Decreased inflammation of your joints and muscles.
- Lowered cholesterol and triglycerides in your bloodstream.
- Aid in the prevention of cancer cell growth.
- Reduced risk of high blood pressure.
- Regulate your food intake, body weight, and metabolism.

Studies have shown that consumption of omega-3 fatty acids, particularly eicosapentaenoic acid (EPA) and docosahexaenoic acid (DHA), greatly increases the strength of the vascular system, improves heart health, and reduces joint inflammation. This is important for athletes who use nonsteroidal anti-inflammatory drugs (NSAIDs) such as aspirin, ibuprofen, and naproxen. Dr. Joseph Maroon, the neurosurgeon for the Pittsburgh Steelers, prompted these studies after years of writing 10 to 20 prescriptions for NSAIDs each day (part of the 70 million each year) and seeing the effect the drugs had on his patients (from improper digestion to gastric hemorrhage) and himself. As an Ironman triathlete, Maroon developed an ulcer from the anti-inflammatory he was using to control his joint pain. After incorporating cod liver oil into his diet, his pain was gone. He put some of his patients on the same regimen and was able to record a 60 percent improvement rate in back pain and inflamma-tion, to the point that some began to cancel surgery and eventually eliminated the use of NSAIDs altogether.[13]

I believe antioxidants are essential as well, particularly for athletes, because without them our bodies would break down. Antioxidants help prevent cellular damage in our bodies from oxidation. Their function is to collect the free radicals that cause damage as a by-product of oxygen use. Free radicals can cause heart and lung damage, skin degeneration, muscular soreness and fatigue, cancer, and a host of other bodily problems. When you live an active lifestyle, your body requires more care. You use more nutrients to support your activity, you lose more minerals and electrolytes because you sweat more, and your body is exposed to more oxidative damage because you breathe more. This is not an argument for sitting on the couch, but rather an acknowledgment that you need to care for your nutrition with more acuity. You can find antioxidants in all sorts of foods:

- Blueberries, oranges, watermelon, tomatoes, grapes, and strawberries.
- Leafy green vegetables, carrots, cranberries, and yellow peppers.
- Nuts, rooibos teas, and the now-famous acai berry.

You will find an abundance of antioxidants with foods from every season, and if you keep in mind the next guideline you will always have them in your diet.

Eat a rainbow of colors. Keep it simple when you shop. Buy a rainbow of foods. The variety will ensure that you are eating balanced meals with complete nutrition. From there, let the recipes in this book help you use those products and allow your body and appetite to stimulate and inspire you further.

Hydrate with pure, filtered water. Our bodies are over 70 percent water, and water is responsible for the function of many of our bodies' cellular and physical operations. As with oxygen, we can't live without water, and also like oxygen, too much of it can lead to problems. When we sweat and breathe, we lose some of the minerals and electrolytes needed to keep our bodies going, especially if we are active. Replenishing with pure, filtered water is crucial to our survival. Unfortunately, some public water supplies are treated with chemicals and additives that destroy the natural composition of water, so it's important to use an environmentally friendly water filtration system instead of tap water when filling up that bottle for your next workout.

For athletes, it is especially important to include electrolytes and minerals in those drinks we hydrate with to help our bodies absorb and replenish nutrients faster and allow us to retain them for later use. There are many manufactured sports drinks and refuelers with artificial electrolytes and minerals, but sometimes they're unnecessary. Nature even has its own perfect sports drink in the form of coconut water. It contains an array of minerals, electrolytes, and sugars that the body can take in rap-

idly. In fact, coconut water so closely matches the body's blood profile that it was used as an intravenous fluid for field trauma during World War II.[14]

Enhance, don't supplement. Why supplement from a factory when you can enhance from nature? Supplements are nothing but substitutes for the real thing. A well-balanced diet can be enhanced by quality choices of EFAs and other specific foods, and this book will show you how to incorporate them into your everyday diet rather than seeking them as something that you need to artificially supply at the end of the day. Remember, staying as close to the plant as you can is the healthiest way to live, and there's nothing further from the plant than an artificial re-creation in a bottle. As legendary triathlete Dave Scott once told me, "If you put crap in, you're going to get crap out!"

Understand your own nutritional requirements. People are like snowflakes; no two are exactly the same. There are many nutritional basics that we can all follow, but from there we branch out in many different directions. As much as we would like to just eat what the person who won the race ate, it is not that simple. Be flexible, listen to the needs of your body, and be willing to respond to those needs when they change. The "Sports Nutrition" chapter of this book contains more specific information on the baseline needs of the athlete's diet.

Make exercise a part of your life, not part of your chore list. This is the core of sustainability. If you don't enjoy whatever you do to exercise, it's not going to last. Life should be active, and an active life should be fun. Sometimes training can be challenging, or even drudgery, but it's all part of a cycle to achieve something greater, to push boundaries. There is something for everyone out there—it does not have to come in the form of a gym membership, a training program, or even running shoes. Keep trying new activities until you find something that you feel improves not only your health and well-being but also how you feel about being active overall.

You Don't Have to Be an Athlete to Have an Active Lifestyle

Not everyone can be, should be, needs to be, or wants to be an athlete. For the purposes of this book, we will consider an athlete as an individual who has a consistent training regimen for the intent of competing within a chosen sport. Within this definition there are varying degrees of intensity that range from the beginner to the age-grouper, the amateur to the professional, but all require a set of sport-specific nutritional considerations for performance improvement and refinement.

I have worked with actors, performers, dancers, yoga instructors, and other individuals who lead very active lives, and used certain aspects of sports nutrition with them, though not to the acute level that I use with those who are training to race. However, even those who are not athletes may need to eat like one. Whether you are someone who goes to the gym

on a regular basis, practices yoga, likes to surf, plays tennis, rides a bike, runs, or swims, or are a parent who chases kids around all day, the bottom line is that you need to eat—and your food, in habit and execution, should support a relationship with the environment, your community, yourself, and whatever type of lifestyle you want to live. Regardless of how you choose to be active, you can still be nourished with seasonal whole foods prepared in simple ways that are healthy and flavorful.

Industrialized living has separated us from a more natural lifestyle, one in which physical activity is a necessity built into each day for a range of purposes such as gardening, hunting, land and house maintenance, and tending to animals. Today, activity comes in many different forms, few of which have to do with self-sufficiency. A nationwide survey found that 70 percent of mothers believe they are similar to an athlete when considering all of their daily activities.[15] Clearly, it is not just athletes who need solid nutritional information, and it's not just chefs who need to know how to cook. Everyone, in my view, needs to understand where food comes from and how to integrate nutrition and cooking into their lives in order to perform their best and live well.

The funny thing is that most athletes I know are some of the worst eaters I come across. Although their bodies may appear to be fit, they are almost always dealing with some kind of nagging injury, a cold or flu, fatigue, muscle pain, or a digestive problem. In many cases, I believe their diets could be at the root of their maladies. Exercise is not an excuse to eat food items that you would not eat otherwise. Those who are not athletes but who are active are at an even greater disadvantage and risk health problems if they have the dietary habits that include refined sugars, carbohydrates, and processed foods. And individuals who are not active in any way face almost certain illness if they eat that way.

What is most important to understand is that the basic elements of eating are the same for everyone. If you are an athlete, you can use the concepts and recipes in this book to enhance the science of sports nutrition to make cooking and eating a simple, enjoyable process that uses whole and natural foods as the source of your nutrition. If you are not an athlete, you can still mine lessons here. Remember, it is a *lifestyle of nutrition* that you need to learn first; you can then apply it so that it supports your particular needs.

The constitution and composition of your body change over time, and so does your ability to participate in sports. But there is no need to learn an entirely new form of eating for each stage of your life. Keep the basics the same and refine the specifics. Is there a better way to look at life than with the idea that to be healthy all you need to do is eat great foods and stay active? As Hippocrates wrote, "Let food be your medicine and let medicine be your food."

Everything we do in life, right down to the simple act of breathing, requires a metabolic action, which means that it needs to be supported by an energy source. Eating should provide your body with an energy source that invigorates you to do the things you need and want regardless of what they are. Food provides our brains with the energy to think, our bodies with the energy to move, and our hearts with the energy to put those things together and be the person that the world needs you to be. No matter what you choose to do, the important thing is how you do it. To bring the best of what you have to offer requires the energy to execute it. Food is the integral part of that energy; our individual activities rely on it.

An active life requires your active participation in your food and your health. Once you gain an understanding of how to build a supportive nutritional lifestyle, you will avoid overeating, you'll promote efficiency, and you will find the timing that will support and enhance your health and daily performance. The point of this book is not to fit you and everyone else into one program that happened to work for me. Its purpose is to introduce you to the techniques that others have used and give you the tools to execute those techniques to make the decisions that support your lifestyle, your palate, and whatever activities you participate in. The recipes are there when you need them, but they should also be a departure point for your own creativity. In the end, the more you know, the less you will have to think about it.

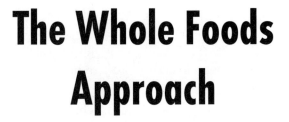

The Whole Foods Approach

Looking at the developed world today, it is easy to forget that we depend entirely on the earth's natural resources for our survival. Long ago, the cultivation of food crops provided societies with the opportunity to remain in one place for yearly planting and harvesting cycles that subsequently established a subsistence form of living. Many of the foods we eat today were derived from the seeds of plants whose ancestors were a variety found in the wild. Although *domestication* is a term normally applied to animals, it was this process of crop selection and cultivation that created the huge variety of farm vegetables grown today. Some of these—the heirlooms—are direct descendants of the plants that were first cultivated, and they maintain the appearances, flavors, and disease and pest resistance of their forebears.

These early gardens were planted to mimic the natural systems of the environment from which they came. The plantings were diverse, proximate, and intermingled for protection and growth support. They were nurtured with natural fertilizers from food, vegetable scraps, plant material, and animal manure, an "organic" approach that helped to strengthen the gene pool while increasing flavor and nutrient content. Although this approach has been largely lost on industrial farms in the pursuit of mechanization and efficiency, small farms today generally still blend and nurture these many elements, which together help to maintain a healthy balance of productivity, diversity, sustainability, and quality.

Understanding Organics

Living with and from the land promotes a relationship that provides a holistic connection between ourselves and our food—and it was the basis for organic agriculture long before the term *organic* existed. Although the organic approach has seen some changes over time, it has always been concerned with taking care of the land so that, in turn, the land will take care of you. It is not just a system of farming but also a philosophy that goes beyond a conventional model of production and profit. This local, seasonal whole foods approach to food production and preparation is one that athletes and active individuals can support because it gives us a connection to our food, satisfies our ecological awareness, alleviates our food-quality concerns, and builds the communities in which we live and work.

But what is organic food, and how does it differ from conventional food? Is it really healthier for you and the planet? The term *organic* was adopted to distinguish a method of food production that does not rely on chemical-based fertilizers or pesticides for crop production, or on artificial hormones and massive quantities of antibiotics for animals.

The large-scale nonorganic agribusiness model of farming in wide use today was developed by the U.S. government shortly after the start of the twentieth century to feed its growing population, as well as to feed hungry people around the world. As the American agricultural model grew from small-scale family farms to larger enterprises, the methods and sources of nutrient input, as well as crop planning and management, needed to change in order to meet the demands of the technology being used. Large farms had to be managed using machinery and systemized methods. What used to be natural, healthy, and diverse techniques of planting a variety of vegetables, fruits, nuts, and flowers within one farm turned into a chemically supported and industrialized form of food production that has done little to cure hunger, let alone sustain our natural resources. If anything, its corporate agenda, land displacement, and political contracts have made things worse. There are many different views on organic agriculture, but to recognize its benefits it is important to understand how conventional methods impact the environment, food quality, and the health of one's body.

Agribusiness vs. Organics

What is generally perceived to be America's bucolic farm system of neatly arranged rows of one type of crop grown over hundreds of acres of land—the system known as monoculture—was in fact developed over the past 100 years or so, and in that time that new system has almost completely replaced the idyllic, small-town, family-style farm of the past. Today's large-scale farms require continuous chemical manipulation and supplementation—from fertilizers and pesticides—to replicate the methods that organic farming on smaller, healthier plots of land relies on. Consequently, as farms grow larger, so does the gap between the ideals surrounding localized organic farming and mass production of food.

Although the agribusiness model was an attempt to grow more food for more people at a faster rate, the health of our environment—and our own health—was unfortunately sacrificed. It's ironic to think that the fertilizers in use today were developed from nitrogen-based bombs used during World War I and that some pesticides—including the ones most commonly used today, such as organophosphates—were modified from nerve gas used in Nazi Germany during World War II.[1] The one thing that was not modified, however, was their impact on all life-forms. Organophosphates are a group of insecticides known to cause neurological defects in animals and humans by interfering with the communication between the body and brain. Other chemical pesticides have also been known to cause respiratory problems, headaches, and skin and eye irritation, as well as cancer, miscarriages, and birth defects. Roundup, the world's best-selling herbicide for the past thirty years, is a commonly used agricultural chemical that can be found in household garages across the country for the control of common weeds. According to Marion Nestle, author of *Safe Food*, it is also "the most common cause of pesticide-related illness among landscape workers and the third most common cause of such illness among ag-

ricultural workers."[2] In 2002 Robert Belle of the National Center for Scientific Research biological station in Roscoff, France, headed a study in which Roundup provoked the first stages of cell division that lead to cancer.[3]

Studies have also shown that once pesticides have been applied, residue can be found in 77 percent of conventional food products.[4] Some of the pesticides are so persistent in the soils where they were used that more than thirty years later they can still be detected in root crops such as carrots, beets, and potatoes, as well as in spinach, lettuce, zucchini, bush beans, and eggplant.[5] The pesticides have also been detected in children whose diets contained fruits and vegetables that organophosphate pesticides had been applied to; they "varied significantly," according to a study completed in 2006, from those who ate organic fruits and vegetables. The collaborative study concluded that "an organic diet provides a dramatic and immediate protective effect against organophosphorus pesticides that are commonly used in agricultural production."[6] Later that same year, Congress enacted the Food Quality Protection Act, which presented the Environmental Protection Agency with the task of overhauling the nation's pesticide laws, especially for infants and children.

What is just as troubling is the fact that these chemicals are not designed to stay within a farm's boundaries. During application or following it, they can get washed or blown into neighboring environments by rain and wind, and drained into the underground water table, subsequently killing animals, polluting waterways, destroying habitat, and creating illness among humans. As early as 1962, biologist Rachel Carson's highly regarded book *Silent Spring* brought to light the potential effects these chemicals—especially the pesticide DDT— were having on the shell formation of bird eggs, the reproductive abilities of mammals, and the survival of marine life. Fortunately, DDT was banned in the United States in 1972, although it was not banned in the United Kingdom until 1984 and is still used in many developing countries today. Despite the ban, DDT residues can still be found in food across North America and northern Europe. As the Environmental Defense Fund noted in a 2005 report, "people throughout the United States still carry DDT and its metabolites in their bodies, 30 years after the pesticide was banned in this country."[7] As recently as 1996, residues of DDT were found in butter, milk, eggs, lamb, potatoes, deep-water fish, and shellfish in the U.K.

Waterways are particularly susceptible to the toxic effects of pesticides, as are the aquatic species that live within them. A 2005 study led by biologist Dr. Rick Relyea, considered to be one of the most extensive surveys of the effects of pesticides on nontarget organisms in an aquatic setting, found that the use of Roundup herbicide in a controlled experiment caused a 70 percent decline in amphibian biodiversity and an 86 percent decline in the total mass of tadpoles; in addition, leopard frog tadpoles and gray tree frog tadpoles were nearly eliminated.[8]

The conventional production of meat and dairy has also become part of this industrial agribusiness—so much so that farms have been replaced by concentrated animal feeding operations (CAFOs). These operations are another by-product of the "get big or get out" model that has chiseled away the number of farmers over the past half-century and created a system of industrial protein production. As with vegetables, the path to efficient mechanized production of animals is through the system of monoculture. On small-scale farms, a variety of animals have contact with humans, fresh soil, air, and sunlight, and their manure is recycled back into the land. In CAFOs, a single breed of livestock is warehoused in confinement with thousands of other like animals without access to a natural environment that would support a healthy diet and humane lifespan. Instead of mimicking the wild foraging of grasses, berries, and bugs in the wild with access to fresh pasture, the animals are fed a diet of conventionally grown grains, corn, and soybeans (and, occasionally, other animal parts) blended with chemical stimulants. In addition, they are regularly injected with hormones and antibiotics to stimulate their appetites, to artificially build muscle, and to protect them from the disease and pestilence created by their confined environment. Clearly, these animals are bred solely for their high meat content in a system based on quantity, not quality.

The hormones used to increase meat production have also been found to be residually present in meat in the marketplace and suspected as a cause for the early onset of puberty in girls, as well as a potential cause of cancer.

As a result, the European Union has banned the importation of hormone-treated beef since 1988. Feeding animals other animal parts was responsible for the rise of mad cow disease, a disease that was initially thought to be confined to dairy and meat stock but was later found to be the cause of a number of deaths in humans. The human version is now known as Variant Creutzfeldt-Jakob disease and by the start of 2009 had claimed 164 lives.

To increase milk production, cows are injected with recombinant bovine growth hormone (rBGH), which has been found to cause substantial increases of instant growth factor (IGF-1) in humans and has been related to breast, colon, and prostate cancer.[9] The rGBH is injected every 14 days for 200 days of a dairy cow's 335-day lactation cycle and dramatically increases milk production. The cows are also fed a dense diet of foods not suited to their digestive system, creating digestive and immune distress that can lead to a disease known as mastitis, an infection within the udder marked by the presence of pus, which is curable with antibiotics. The antibiotics and pus from mastitis have been found in market-ready milk, which has led to the ban of rBGH in Canada and Europe.

The agribusiness model of confining a large herd of animals in one place also results in a high concentration of waste. Its effect on the environment and the people living in the farms' proximity has its own set of polluting and destructive issues. Once created, the waste needs to be handled and managed. I remember my first trip driving across the country. Shortly after crossing the Colorado border with the windows down and the plains breezes blowing, I was suddenly accosted by a putrid smell. "What is that?" I asked my traveling companion. "Smells like shit," he said. As we crested a hill, there were undulating swaths of black visible in the distance amid the brown landscape of the Colorado flatlands. Before long it was clear that these "swaths" were beef cattle and that the undulations in the landscape were created by manure. The sight of this was nothing short of appalling. I saw for myself how the nation's cattle were allowed to live in the waste that surrounded them.

The favored method of dealing with all this manure is to use it as a fertilizer by spraying it on farm fields. However, because thousands of tons are produced weekly and are repeatedly applied to the same fields, a surplus results. The excess manure sometimes enters streams and lakes, contaminating them and destroying aquatic life, as well as rendering the waterways unfit for human use in any form. Air-quality concerns accompany the deposition of all that manure for those who are unfortunate enough to live close to where these herds are raised.

The manufacturing side of the growth and preparation of meat and produce has its own set of additives designed to ward off contamination, insect damage, and spoilage and encourage ripening. The use of chemicals, irradiation, and water for the final stages of transporting these products to the marketplace is a study all its own. Add to all of this the problems of swine flu, meat recalls, and foodborne illnesses, and it is clear that our food system has gone awry. Consumers must remain the driving force in determining how our food is grown and delivered to the markets, guided by reestablishing our connection to the earth and the natural cultivation of the food we eat.

Genetically Modified Organisms

An additional component of the industrialized food system is the use of genetically modified organisms (GMOs), whose DNA has been modified by the insertion of a gene or genes from another organism. The World Health Organization defines them as "organisms in which the genetic material (DNA) has been altered in a way that does not occur naturally."[10] GMOs have a number of applications in pharmaceutical drugs and medical research and are most abundantly used in agriculture. A number of GMOs on the market today have been developed with genetic traits that provide a resistance to pests, tolerance to pesticides, or assist in the processing of food products as additives to improve their quality. Field crops such as Bt-corn, Bt-sweet corn, Roundup Ready soybeans, and Roundup Ready corn are common GMO crops.

Due to the widespread plantings of single crops over large acreages—the monoculture model mentioned earlier—insects that feed on certain plant varieties have the ability to proliferate and destroy large amounts of that crop. The corn borer is one of those insects. Continued application of chemical pesticides did not kill all of the corn borers; those that

lived developed a resistance to the chemicals. In response, biotech companies engineered the corn itself to produce a pesticidal protein called Bt-toxin so when the corn borer attempted to eat the corn, the borer would die. Subsequently, Bt-corn, sold in supermarkets, was registered as an insecticide.

In the case of Roundup Ready crops, these were genetically engineered to be resistant to the spraying of the Roundup pesticide, as it kills everything else around it. Today, 90 percent of the soybeans grown in the United States are Roundup Ready. All are used for human consumption either directly—in food products like tofu, protein powders, and recovery drinks—or indirectly, when they enter the food chain as animal feed for meat production.

The issue of safety with regard to modified crops is controversial even within the U.S. Food and Drug Administration (FDA). According to the 1992 FDA policy on genetically modified foods, "The agency is not aware of any information showing that foods derived by these new methods differ from other foods in any meaningful or uniform way."[11] This means that the FDA officially considers these foods to be safe. However, dissension among FDA employees regarding this policy has been made public. Dr. Louis Pribyl's "Comments on Biotechnology Draft Document," dated February 27, 1992, states, "There is a profound difference between the types of unexpected effects from traditional breeding and genetic engineering." And in response to the *Federal Register* document prepared by the FDA, "Statement of Policy: Foods from Genetically

Modified Plants" (1992), FDA compliance officer Dr. Linda Kahl noted that "the document is trying to force the ultimate conclusion that there is no difference between foods modified by genetic engineering and foods modified by traditional breeding. . . . The process of genetic engineering and traditional breeding are different, and according to technical experts in the agency, they lead to different risks."

As a result, the FDA made it the responsibility of the food producer to ensure that its foods are safe when delivered to the marketplace, ultimately leaving the biotech companies to police themselves and their own products. According to Phil Angell, the director of corporate communication for Monsanto, the company that developed and distributes Roundup, "Monsanto should not have to vouchsafe the safety of biotech food. Our interest is in selling as much of it as possible. Assuring its safety is the FDA's job."[12]

The upshot of this disclaimer of responsibility is that the fox is guarding the henhouse and the duty of determining the safety of food rests largely on the consumer. This task is made more difficult by the fact that the products containing GMOs—which amount to about 70 percent of the food products in America's stores—do not have to be labeled as such.

The biggest risk factor in GMO foods is the potential transference of modified food genes into our bodies. Numerous fetal studies on mice have confirmed that ingested DNA can enter the developing fetus through the placenta.[13] There is also mounting anecdotal evidence on the effects these crops may have on the animals that are fed hormones and GMOs. In his groundbreaking book on GMO foods, *Genetic Roulette,* Jeffrey M. Smith writes, "About two dozen farmers report that GM [genetically modified] corn varieties caused their pigs or cows to become sterile, 71 shepherds say that 25 percent of their sheep died from grazing on Bt cotton plants, and others say that cows, water buffaloes, chickens, and horses also died from eating GM crops."[14]

Avoiding GMO foods can be challenging but not impossible. Following the credos outlined in this book will help you avoid them. Using the GMO food sources list found in the back of the book, and checking www.responsibletechnology.org for updates to this list, will keep you informed.

Note, however, that foods made specifically for athletes often contain these additives. It is important to read the labels of the ones you choose. To help avoid GMOs, look for supplements that are made with raw ingredients and without additives (see Chapter 4).

Choosing Organics

Society today does not have to return to a subsistence form of living to ensure the quality of our food and prevent the effects that the agribusiness model has had on it and the environment. Our society does, however, need to recognize this impact. Not only have we lost some of our natural resources but, over the past fifty years, there has also been a decline in the nutrient content of conventionally grown vegetables and fruits by up to 40 percent.[15] Vegetables that are grown on organic farms as well as the animals that are raised on them feed and live off the nutrients and minerals provided by the earth and its natural processes. This assimilation provides a higher degree of nutrient content in crops and meat products. Studies have shown that organic crops contain significantly higher levels of minerals, iron, magnesium, phosphorus, and vitamin C in addition to much lower levels of heavy metals and nitrates than conventionally grown crops.[16] A recent study found that organic tomatoes contained an average of 1,938 milligrams of iron each versus 1 milligram for nonorganic tomatoes, and that organic lettuce contained 516 milligrams of iron, compared to just 9 milligrams for the nonorganic variety (see Figure 2.1).[17]

Having a finely tuned body is paramount to athletes, and any loss of nutrients can affect

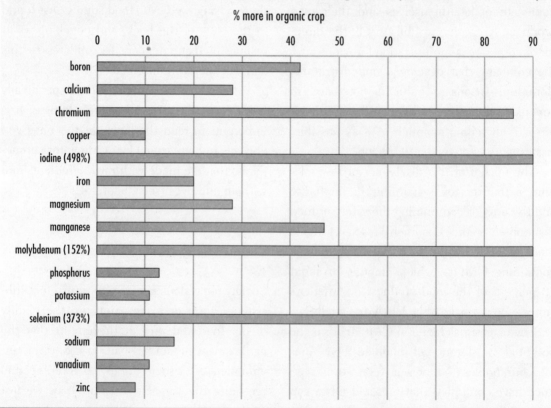

FIGURE 2.1: Mean percentage additional mineral content in organic compared to conventional crops

Source: "Variations in Mineral Content in Vegetables," Soil Society of America Proceedings 13 (1998): 380–384. Used by permission of the Soil Society of America.

performance. As you will see in this book, a diet based on high-quality food sources promotes a healthy, disease-free, and athletically supported life. Health concerns caused by poor nutrition are not limited to cancer, diabetes, and heart problems; they can also encompass hair loss, dental caries, back problems, and other injuries that are not specifically trauma related. Three-time Olympic swimmer Erik Vendt consumes only organic foods and credits this diet for his return to competitive form, greater energy, increased muscle mass, and better overall health as compared to a previous diet based on foods that were not holistic to his training. Elite endurance waterman Jamie Mitchell also believes in eating only organic foods to boost his performance, stating flatly, "Organic is the way to go."[18] Athletes demand a lot from their bodies, and attention to nutrition boosts performance exponentially. Six-time Ironman champion triathlete Dave Scott refers to this care and feeding of an athlete's body as the "unknown element" and credits it with his athletic success. It is the responsibility of every athlete to always keep in mind that healthy organic food is linked to the earth, and the earth requires our vigilant stewardship of its resources if we expect it to continue to perform. This is why our lifestyle must support our nutrition if, in turn, we want our nutrition to support our natural resources.

There are many reasons why people choose to purchase organic food. As the public recognition of the inferior quality of conventional food products has increased, the demand for organic food has risen steadily. Since 1990 the market share of organic foods has grown by about 20 percent per year. Total sales now reach the billions of dollars. Conventional food producers recognized the appeal of organic foods some years ago and began to mislabel their products to capitalize on the growing organic market. In response, private and state organic certification programs began in the 1970s and 1980s to ensure organic properties, but it was not until 1990 that the federal Organic Foods Production Act was passed and guidelines began to be established for the National Organic Program (NOP). The National Organic Standards Board (NOSB) was established as the program's governing body and in 1992 began to set regulations for the production and handling of agricultural products aimed at the marketplace. However, opposition from agribusiness companies—which feared that organic certification would create an unfair market distinction—impeded the implementation of the NOP guidelines for ten years. The big food companies had reason to fear; consumers began to understand that organics were worth the distinction. The NOP guidelines set certain production standards that organic foods and their ingredients needed to meet for specific labeling requirements. As a result, these standards provided consumers with reliability, trust, and quality they could count on.

The guidelines were an extension of the practices that were already being used by farmers who understood the connection among land management, food, people, and the earth. The guidelines gave consumers the ability to differentiate quality and make conscious choices about what they ate. Under the guidelines, vegetables are grown without the use of chemical pesticides or fertilizers, and without the contamination and addition of human or industrial waste or GMOs. Livestock are raised without the consistent and sub-therapeutic use of growth hormones, antibiotics, or other drugs. The food that is fed to the animals similarly must be produced under the same NOP guidelines, without being treated with any drugs whatsoever. Vegetables, fruits, chickens, and so on must also be free of food additives, ionizing radiation, chemical ripening agents, and genetically modified organisms. The guidelines also state that organic products are to be raised under ecologically based practices to enhance soil fertility by using decomposed organic materials and nutrients—known as compost—along with cover crops that actually capture and use nutrients from the air, such as nitrogen, and put those nutrients back into the soil. In addition, animals and plants should be rotated each year to prevent depletion of the soil nutrients so the land does not lose topsoil or become overgrazed and destroyed. Also, vegetables are planted in companionship and intermixed with other plants as part of the old system of natural, biological cultivation that is able to control pests, weeds, and diseases as well as to prevent widespread crop failure.

In the United States, federal legislation defines three levels of labeling for products that are organic. These requirements are "national standards that apply to raw, fresh and unprocessed products that contain organic in-gredients and are based on the percentage of organic ingredients in a product."[19] Products made entirely with certified organic ingredients and by certified organic methods can be labeled "100 percent organic." Products made with at least 95 percent organic ingredients can use the word "organic." These two categories may also display the U.S. Department of Agriculture (USDA) organic seal. The third category—products containing a minimum of 70 percent organic ingredients—can be labeled "made with organic ingredients" but cannot use the USDA seal. In addition, products may display the logo of the certification body, such as the NOFA (Northeast Organic Farming Association), OTA (Oregon Tilth Association), or CCOF (California Certified Organic Farmers), that approved them.

There is also a category for farmers and handlers who sell less than $5,000 worth of organic agricultural products per year. Provided they have the proper paperwork to support them, farmers in this group are exempt from certification but cannot label their products as certified organic.

Over the years the word *organic* has gone from function to fashion, and to a form of industrialization itself. Today, *organic* and the USDA label can be seen on food products—produce, meats, dairy foods, beverages—as well as detergents, household cleaners, hair and skin products, clothes, bedding, mattresses, yard care, and pest management products. There are even restaurants that have been certified organic. Chances are if you're looking for a product to be organic, you can find it.

As a result, some of the organic practices used today have been industrialized and employ similar agricultural practices to their conventional counterparts, such as monoculture plantings on massive acreage and USDA-approved "organic" chemicals. However, within all of this still remains the purity of the initial movement and the farm systems that preceded it. Today, small farmers are going "beyond organic" by creating ecological and sustainable food systems that transcend the standards set forth by the organic certification laws.

Eating with the Seasons

"Eating seasonally makes sense," says adventure racer, triathlete, and ultrarunner Terri Schneider, who shops regularly at her local farmers' market.[20] She, along with many other high-performance athletes, recognizes that the quality of the food she eats is critical to the refinement of her performance. Purchasing the freshest food available is a natural response to this pursuit. Packing in somewhere around 3,000 calories a day can be an effort for some athletes, and others may need to consume more than twice that amount. One of the problems with consciously planning your calorie intake is lack of time and forethought. Between work, family, and other commitments, finding the time to train can be difficult enough without having to think about—let alone prepare—one's meals.

The result becomes a quick fix of the same foods, and a lot of them tend to be processed, containing refined carbohydrates and sugars, even if they do have organic labels on them. My solution to this quandary is to eat with the seasons. By doing so, you will easily incorporate nutrient-dense foods, limit your time spent thinking about what to eat, and automatically default to making the most of what is "naturally" readily available to you.

For athletes such as myself, eating is right up there with running on trails under a green canopy of leaves or surfing a glassy wave at sunset. In fact, sometimes I think I love to be active simply because I love to eat. Regardless of whether eating is the point of training or the other way around, athletic endeavors require nutritional support—and during competition you need an even more specific approach to food.

Whether your body uses 1,500 or 6,000 calories per day, providing your body with this energy can become a monotonous experience. Eating the same foods, bought from the same market and prepared in the same way, day after day, is a common pitfall of many athletes. During his fourteen years as a National Hockey League goalie, Mike Richter learned that "athletes get everything from superstitious to routine and as a result end up eating the same meal every day before competition and training. You can get away with this for a little while," he notes, "but eventually something will break down."[21] Not only is the repetition boring, but it fails to address the basic nutritional principle that you should eat a variety of foods to provide the cells in your body with all of the nutrients needed to sustain energy requirements and overall health. As Dan Benardot writes in his book, *Nutrition for Serious Athletes,* "It is clear that monotonous intakes of this type will eventually lead to some degree of malnutrition and, for the athlete, some loss of performance potential."[22]

There also is no one secret recipe that successful athletes have found to work and that they eat over and over. Combinations of different foods have synergistic reactions that benefit different types of bodily functions, and athletes need them all. "You need to diversify your foods from different sources and different types to continue to perform," notes Richter. Failure to do so can eventually lead to health problems, injuries, and athletic impediments.

I have seen this happen with athletes—from professional to amateur—and active individuals alike. A client came to me two months before an event for which she had been training for almost a year because she feared her body might not hold up until race day. I asked her to keep a food diary for three days. She returned with one day's entries and a notation of a few substitutes; she basically ate the same things every day. Moreover, what she ate primarily came in packages, including the majority of her vegetables, along with a number of the latest and greatest supplements. When we discussed her daily energy levels and training schedule, she mentioned that she was always fatigued, was unmotivated for back-to-back days of training, and began to skip her brick workouts (consecutive swim-bike or bike-run workouts) because she could not get through them. She eventually developed a nagging injury, which she treated with medication, and had headaches at night.

Not only did she need some nutrient-packed food, she also needed to add variety to her diet and make some adjustments to the times when she ate. Luckily, she lived in an area where there were farmers' markets every week. I instructed her to buy what was there, talk to the farmers, and concentrate on selecting organic foods as often as possible. I assured her that if she could learn to listen to her body, it would guide her. She took my advice, and soon after, her diet and mental and physical disposition began to change dramatically—so much so that the injury stopped nagging her, the medication became unnecessary, and her energy returned. Best of all, she took more than ten minutes off her race time! Although she did not think of herself as a good cook, eating with the seasons was a simple way to allow the ingredients on hand to do the work for her.

This client's success is not unusual. In fact, her results can be true for everyone, athlete or otherwise, because they come from the simple rule of always eating a variety of seasonal foods. By following the seasonal progression of fruits and vegetables, you can easily achieve a nutritional balance in your food supply that optimizes health and athletic performance.

Eating with the seasons means buying meat and produce at a time during the year when it is naturally growing in your local region. I encourage you to buy organic food as much as possible, though not if that means the organic food has traveled great distances. Today, chain-store supermarkets and even Walmart stores offer organic "fresh" foods but, as detailed below, fresh is not fresh if the food has been shipped a great distance.

My first choice for food shopping is always the farmers' market. I get to smell, touch, feel, and, quite often, taste everything I want before I buy it. Plus, I get to contribute to my local economy, meet the people that have grown the food, ask questions, watch their children grow, and, in some ways, feel that I am part of the process. Just being at the farmers' market makes me feel healthy.

Agriculturally, seasons are defined by frost dates, when the temperature falls below freezing. The first frost marks the start of fall, when only cooler crops—broccoli, cabbages, Brussels sprouts, apples, pears—can survive. When a long stretch of freezing occurs, winter has arrived, and it is time for potatoes, winter squash, carrots, onions, Jerusalem artichokes, parsnips, and turnips. The last frost date of the winter months marks the time when spring produce will begin to mature. Look for peas, asparagus, lettuce, and all kinds of greens at this time. This is also the time when summer crops are planted; they will begin to be harvested within six weeks (green beans) to nine weeks (tomatoes).

Although it is mainly fruits and vegetables that are seasonal, you should also consider fish and meats seasonally. Fish migrate during different seasons, and many are specific to local waters. Most farmers' markets align themselves with fishmongers; if not, look to your local seafood shop to instruct you on what is freshest. Meats—lamb, chicken, beef—and raw dairy are excellent in spring, when the animals have been grazing on fresh grasses and contain beneficial nutrients such as omega-3s, whereas pork is best in the fall after feasting on the scraps of summer's vegetable bounty.

When you buy from farmers' markets your money goes directly into the hands of the person or family that owns, works, and devotes precious time to the farm. By eliminating the middlemen, your food expenditures can decrease up to 40 percent, depending on where you shop.[23] Some farms have organized Community Supported Agriculture (CSA) programs whereby you prepay a certain membership fee at the beginning of the farming season. After that, you drop by the market each week and pick up your box of freshly harvested goodies. In this case you don't even have to choose; the farmers do it for you. Not only that, but an added time-saver would be to join with some friends and rotate each week who picks them up—carpooling at its best! The products available at these farms can range from meats, raw dairy products, and vegetables to value-added products such as jams, honey, and bread. Combined with a monthly trip to a health or specialty store for bulk items, such programs drastically limit the time you will spend shopping for food.

Farmers' markets can be found all over the country. In the past, most operated only during the prime summer and fall months. Today, however, in many areas of the country they open in the early spring and continue into the late fall. These markets used to carry only fruits and vegetables, but today most include vendors offering baked goods, meats, cheeses, and fish. Even these items have their season, and by continuing to shop at the farmers' markets you will naturally become accustomed to and eventually begin to expect and look forward to items that are on their way! Living on the eastern seaboard, I know that spring is here when the asparagus are sprouting, summer is on its way when the strawberries begin to appear and is full on when the sunflowers are in bloom, fall has arrived when the apples make their way to market, and winter is near when Brussels sprouts are available. Even in the heart of New York City there are farmers' markets and co-op gardens. While traveling throughout the country I have found local produce available almost everywhere.

Also, talk with your local produce managers in the larger markets, and tell them that you would like to see more local items in the store. You can visit www.truefoodnow.org and www.localharvest.org to locate the farmers' markets, CSAs, and health food stores in your area (see the "Resources" chapter in this book). Every county also has a local extension office that will provide this type of information; it can be found in the county government section of your phone book under the community college heading.

As you frequent farmers' markets, you will begin to note that fruits and vegetables grow during different seasons in different regions. Almost nothing is available year-round. For instance, tomatoes and other fruits don't grow in the Northeast during winter, and indeed most fresh produce can be in limited supply. To keep a variety of vegetables in your diet in colder climates, frozen vegetables are preferable for their nutrient retention over fresh, conventional, and, sometimes, organic produce that has been grown far away and shipped over long distances. Frozen vegetables are harvested at their peak and almost immediately flash-frozen at temperatures of 30 degrees below zero. This quick freezing maintains the high nutritive value of the product without the use of artificial preservatives by slowing down its chemical changes. Barbara Klein, a food scientist at the University of Illinois at Urbana, did a comparative study of fresh and frozen vegetables. After a year of frozen storage, green beans had twice as much vitamin C content as fresh green beans that were in a refrigerator for three days. Klein states that almost 58 percent of the vitamin C content in unfrozen green beans is lost after three days.[24]

You can freeze produce at home during the summer when an abundance of it is available. Blueberries, for example, are loaded with antioxidants, freeze well, and are great for smoothies. Buy them in bulk and freeze them on a cookie sheet lined with parchment paper. Purchasing a home dehydrator and using it to dry fruits like apples, pineapple, tomatoes, and peaches at temperatures below 118 degrees is another way to preserve food and its nutrients. Low-temperature dehydration retains all of the vital enzymes, minerals, and vitamins that the food has to offer. Once dried, the foods can be used in a variety of ways and also enjoyed raw.

There are many resources for using a dehydrator and preserving the raw nutrients of food (see the "Resources" chapter).

Another great way to preserve nutrients is through a process known as lacto-fermentation, or pickling. This can also be done at home. Almost all vegetables can be pickled, and adding your own herbs and spices lets you be creative and provides you with the variety you need in your diet throughout the year. If you instead buy pickled products at a store, it is important to choose ones that are raw. The majority of foods that are bottled and packaged go through a pasteurization process that kills all of the beneficial nutrients, enzymes, probiotics, and amino acids that you are trying to preserve.

Eating with the seasons means getting not only peak flavor but also the highest nutritional value a fresh product has to offer. Soon after vegetables are harvested in the field, their nutrients begin to diminish. Once harvested, vegetables can no longer produce their enzymatic reactions because they are not being supplied with a source of energy from the plant. Their attempt at compensating is to utilize the remaining nutrients within. Vitamin C, an important antioxidant, diminishes especially quickly; for example, kale loses 1 to 5 percent of its vitamin C content *per hour* post-harvest, while peas, broccoli, and green beans lose 20 to 40 percent and spinach 90 percent within three days of harvest. Folic acid, which is vital in amino acid metabolism, shows a similar loss in most vegetables, at a rate of 50 to 70 percent.[25]

Sara Hanafin, a registered dietitian at the Boulder Center for Sports Medicine in Colorado, says the best produce comes from farmers' markets offering food picked the same day it is sold. If you can't eat it that same day, she advises using the produce within a day or two.[26] The recipes in this book will help you follow this advice.

Consider the impact that transportation has on organically grown fresh produce purchased in large supermarkets. Produce that is found in chain supermarkets was, most likely, harvested *two to three weeks* prior to purchase and may even have been grown in and shipped from another country. According to the Worldwatch Institute, the average distance food travels from grower to market is between 1,500 and 2,500 miles.[27] In addition to these products having lost a large portion of their nutrients, vegetables that are shipped over long distances are picked early, sprayed to delay ripening, and require an abundance of fossil fuels for transport and processing. Eating locally reduces your exposure to these chemicals and helps you avoid nutrient-deficient foods.

There's another benefit to eating seasonally and locally, direct from the farmer: the risk of food contamination dramatically decreases. In 2006, *E. coli* contamination of fresh spinach killed three people in the United States. This spinach, which had been irrigated with water contaminated with cattle feces containing the *E. coli* bacterium, was the product of a 50-acre industrial monoculture farm in San Benito County, California. Obviously, you must wash all raw foods in fresh water before consumption, but in my experience your exposure to contaminants is much lower with locally sourced vegetables.

Cooking also becomes a much easier process when vegetables are at their peak. As Gary Danko, one of the country's top chefs and winner of a James Beard Foundation "Best Chef" award, points out, "If you are using ingredients grown in season, you're going to have the maximum amount of flavor those products can deliver."[28] There is no need to add a lot of ingredients to have meals that taste good. Remember, why cook what you can eat raw?

Let the season, as well as your body, dictate how you cook. Do you feel like eating a heavy beef stew in the middle of summer and watermelon in winter? Probably not. Cook light during the summer by eating lots of fresh crisp salads, steamed veggies and fish, and a seasonal progression of fruits. Autumn is a transition time when corn, mushrooms, garlic, fennel, and apples begin to fill the stands at the farmers' markets. Winter calls for the heartiest foods, such as beets, winter squash, rutabagas, Jerusalem artichokes, and potatoes; and spring completes the cycle with asparagus, strawberries, fava beans, and new greens. By following the seasons you will also find yourself trying new foods and preparing them in different ways. Maintaining your own vegetable-and-herb garden will allow you to enjoy seasonally fresh produce and give you a better appreciation of caring for the earth.

Eating should be a reward, but it also should supply fuel for your muscles' hard work.

Whether we are active for pleasure or because we are training in a specific sport, there is one rule we all must obey: energy expenditure requires the right foods for energy replacement. Eating with the seasons will increase your health and your connection with the environment and will make whatever aerobic activity you are doing the glorious experience it is meant to be.

Native Foods Are Your Best Prevention

The term *diet* has unfortunately come to be defined as what people should *not* eat to achieve specific goals. These goals may be weight loss, weight gain, or disease prevention (combating high cholesterol, for example). To me, however, diet is a reflection of one's lifestyle. As Geneen Roth states, "We eat the way we live. What we do with food, we do in our lives. Eating is a stage upon which we act out our beliefs about ourselves."[29] You must maintain a diet that sustains both your individual health and the health of our planet. It is obvious by looking at the incidence of disease and obesity today that contemporary "diets" based on the perspectives of a few individuals using short-term research and that include a host of processed foods do not work. A diet based on the seasonal availability of local whole foods does.

Dr. Weston Price, a dentist and nutritionist who headed the research section of the American Dental Association from 1914 to 1923, was among the first to discover the difference between the health of individuals living in isolated areas consuming indigenous foods and that of communities living within modern society whose diets were based on processed foods. Based on his diverse travels to different corners of the world, his conclusions were uniformly clear. In his book *Nutrition and Physical Degeneration,* published in 1939, he described how people whose diets were based on local natural foods enjoyed long lives that were virtually devoid of commonly found diseases, whereas those whose diets consisted of refined carbohydrates, sugars, and other industrialized processed foods displayed a veritable cross section of the diseases found today.

Studies of centenarians—individuals living beyond 100 years of age—include the people of the Caucasus in Soviet Russia (Abkhazians), the Karakorum Range (Hunzas), the Arctic (Eskimos), Crete (Cretans), Japan (Okinawans), and the Ecuadorian Andes (Vilcabambas). The lives of these people were in no way sedentary, but they lived without the processed and refined foods that have come to be synonymous with modern societies. In fact, some remarkable athletes with elite showings in long-distance running have hailed from the Tarahumara Indians of northern Mexico and the Kalenjin tribe of Kenya, two societies that follow a diet based on native foods without the scientific knowledge of sports nutrition.

The whole foods diets that lead to such successful outcomes and long lifetimes are ultimately quite simple. The majority are plant-based. They consist of plenty of green vegetables or seaweeds, of which a good portion are eaten raw or lightly cooked. Meat and fish are only occasionally eaten, depending on geography—the farther inland, the less fish; the closer to sea, the fewer other forms of meat—and when meat is consumed, it comes from wild game or animals that are free-roaming and have grazed on fresh grasses. The fish that is eaten has been caught in the wild, not farm raised. Most followers of a traditional whole foods diet also incorporated the organs of those animals into their diet in some way, quite often raw. Dairy products from pastured raised livestock, including raw milk, cheeses, and butter, are also often a part of these native diets. Whole grains and legumes such as corn, wheat, quinoa, buckwheat, rye, and beans were generally soaked, sprouted, and/or fermented, then freshly ground for breads, tortillas, or porridge.

Virtually all cultures that subsist on traditional foods use some form of fermentation, be it for dairy, vegetables, grains, or an animal source such as cod liver oil. The result is a diet that is rich in omega-3s, live enzymes, and minerals. The proportions might break down loosely to an average of 55 percent fats, 15 percent protein, and 30 percent carbohydrates. Interestingly enough, two cultures that greatly deviate from this average are the Kalenjin and Tarahumara. Their diets consist of a much higher proportion of carbohydrates, upward of 70 percent, with fats and proteins being closer to 15 percent each. Not surprisingly, these proportions are very similar to the composition of an aerobic diet and supportive of the long-distance running that is central to each of these cultures.

It is one thing to examine a group of people, their diet, and their health and begin to extrapolate conclusions using those observations. However, what Dr. Price and others have done is to examine the reversion of disease and illness when an individual transitions from a contemporary diet of processed foods to one that is more natural and organic. This concept goes as far back as the Tang dynasty, when physician Sun Ssu Mo in his book *Precious Recipes* stated, "A truly good physician first finds the cause of illness, and having found that, he tries to cure it by food. Only when food fails does he prescribe medication."[30] My own experience supports this observation. I believe that the majority of disease that exists today is directly linked to our consumption of highly processed foods. Eliminating processed foods from one's diet allows the body to display its amazing ability for recovery and regeneration. In the athletes I work with, I have seen that switching to a whole foods diet leads to an increase in performance, shorter recovery times, and, most important, the prevention of injuries.

Most individuals in the United States base their diet on the conveniences of processed food and an agricultural system that reflects an industrial business model. The busy athlete is no exception, and a transition to a whole foods diet might therefore seem very difficult. However, to make such a change only requires information, support, and accessibility to proper foods. Thankfully, the principles of organic agriculture and traditional diets have not been lost, and with the local food supply available in farmers' markets today it is easy to follow a sustainable lifestyle that will lead to better nutrition and health. The recipes in this book have been designed to support and nurture this nutritional approach. Because all of us are part of nature's cycle, we can easily become part of it again.

Sometimes a change in lifestyle requires a more intimate process, a period of time in which the body can heal, realign itself, reestablish its connection to the earth, and recreate its relationship with food. For centuries, fasting has been used as a method to allow the innate wisdom and healing technologies of the body to do this. Today, fasting can be utilized for the same purposes along with the time to evaluate one's current nutritional habits and lifestyle. Methods of fasting range from consuming solely water to the consumption of specific foods. What I have found to be the most effective is a weeklong consumption of vegetable and fruit juices combined with detoxification adjuncts, such as herbs, minerals, and clay, as well as yoga, massage, and personal quiet time, to assist the body in cleansing the digestive tract. As Stephen Harrod Buhner describes the process in his book *The Fasting Path,* the body "uses its energy during a fast not for digesting food but for cleansing the body of accumulated toxins and healing any parts of it that are ill. As a fast progresses, the body consumes everything it can that is not essential to bodily functioning. This includes bacteria, viruses, fibroid tumors, waste products in the blood, any buildup around the joints and stored fat."[31] Once your body has been cleaned out and then fed with whole foods in their unrefined state, it will tell you thereafter that it wants and needs those foods.

I have witnessed almost miraculous healing effects take place in individuals who have given their body and digestive system a rest and an opportunity to heal. I have also known people who have made lasting modifications to their nutritional intake—modifications that are not based on flash-in-the-pan diets. A temporary departure from regular meals provides an opportunity to reflect on one's habits, the types of foods we consume, how much of those foods we eat at one sitting, and the overall difference in how we feel and perform.

Along with being an elite endurance runner and author, Bernd Heinrich is a renowned biologist. He had noted that animals in the wild fast when they are ill as part of their innate healing wisdom.[32] I have seen this in my dogs when their bodies are fighting off some kind of sickness. They may not have the intellectual development and understanding to make a conscious choice, but they are responding to their natural proclivities. Keep in mind that I do not see fasting as a mechanism for weight loss on its own, but a convergence of necessity among the body, the mind, the spirit, and proper timing to aid in the facilitation of healing.

Despite the prevalence of the industrial food system, we have not reached a nutritional dead end and we have not run out of options. Living our lives with nature provides a sense of humility in accepting that bigger does not necessarily mean better when it comes to our food supply.

We must continue to appreciate and develop an understanding of the food that is the fuel that drives our bodies to perform and to stay healthy. When we can make learning about the benefits of, shopping for, and cooking with organic, whole, raw foods part of our lifestyle, this nutritional approach will naturally blend into our schedules and become second nature.

3

Eating Made Easy

Like anything in life, preparing good meals requires the right tools, some practice, a willingness to learn, and, most important, the balance and discipline it takes to make these factors work for you. Add to this a diet based on an understanding of organics, "eating with the seasons," a whole foods approach, and using food instead of supplements to maintain health, and you will find yourself guided by subconscious intuition and what your body is telling you it needs. However, none of this works unless you participate in your own buying, preparing, and cooking, along with recognizing the importance of the foods you eat. To many people, cooking seems an overwhelming task, but it doesn't have to be. Food can be easy to prepare, and the time you spend cooking can help you find the balance and connection to yourself, your family, your community, and the natural world. And, of course, the food you prepare provides the fuel to support your endeavors. "Cooking your own food makes a huge difference in your athletic performance," says Mike Richter, the retired New York Rangers goalie who, during his career, did his own shopping and prepared his own meals because he knew how important it was to his success.[1]

Eating for an Active Lifestyle

Eating should not complicate life. It should enhance life's quality, not only from a nutritional standpoint but also from a social one. Some of our fondest memories come from meals cooked and shared with family and friends. There is a need to schedule your training, gym, and workout times, but your food shopping and eating should be part of the natural flow of your life.

If you want good, wholesome food to be convenient, you have to make it that way. The commercially prepared foods that are readily available and "convenient" will not support your daily performance in a sustainable way. Your food consumption is important for your entire life, not just to support your athletic pursuits, and there is simply no substitute for real foods and traditional cooking methods.

One of the most important lessons in adapting a successful nutritional strategy for an active lifestyle—from recreational running to competitive racing—is for the athlete or individual to spend time getting in touch with his or her body and its subsequent needs. It is a process that requires continual adjustments and being open to trying new things and exploring new ideas. After more than 15 years of perfecting my nutrition and incorporating it into my life, I am still learning new methods and discovering new foods. To be proficient at anything requires patience, practice, and repetition, but it's always worth the effort, and the more you do it, the less work it will require. As with any workout routine, maintaining your daily nutrition, learning about what your body needs—and does not need—and integrating these steps into your busy life will pay its dividends in better performance.

The cooking credos I identify are the concepts that will help guide you in the execution of a master plan to eat well in a sustainable way. The micro aspects of this nutritional framework, such as serving sizes, when to eat, and how much to eat, will become part of your intuition as you practice these concepts and consume a better-quality diet grounded in whole foods. In my experience with many athletes, calculating numbers and quantities of calories, along with weighing food for portioning, can be a short-lived endeavor. An athletic life aimed at maximum performance has different requirements than one for someone who wants to lose weight or begin a fitness routine. For the various lifestyles of individuals who are trained athletes and those who merely want to be fit, the next two chapters will present guidelines for general nutrition (Chapter 4) and sports nutrition (Chapter 5). However, the following guidelines apply to both the endurance athlete and the gym-going soccer mom.

Align Yourself with Your Food and Your Community

Making healthy eating a seamless part of your lifestyle begins with the process of bringing yourself, your food, and your community together. Eating seasonally and choosing locally grown whole foods are where the lifestyle of nutrition truly begins. It is the most important of my nutrition credos, and understanding and following it will naturally guide you into the rest of them. Although it might seem easy to be told what and how to eat, long-term results and consistency come from creating a system that will be the foundational answer to any food challenges you may face.

Understand Labels and Packaging

Entering a supermarket today can be a daunting task if you are trying to eat well and live a healthy lifestyle. According to the Food Market Institute, in 2006 there were approximately 45,000 food products on the shelves, and all of them had a label.[2] The majority of these foods are highly processed and contain large amounts of refined sugars and carbohydrates. Moreover, many of them also contain corn-based by-products as well as ingredients from genetically modified organisms (GMOs). This majority, by the way, also includes the "natural foods" aisle, where many people get tricked into thinking the products are "safe," especially for those who are vegetarians. In large part, a society is defined by its food consumption and its relationship to the environment. For an understanding of our consumer-oriented society, you need only read the labels that appear on the tens of thousands of "convenient" food products that are the stock-in-trade of every major supermarket chain in the country.

The labels on packaged foods have become the main source of information for what we put into our bodies. We should not rely on them to the extent we do for quality, safety, or nutrient content, or use them as a guide for what we eat. However, most of us do not even take the time to read these labels and would be unable to understand them if we did. Gone are the days prior to high-fructose corn syrup, FD&C dyes, enriched flours, partially hydrogenated oils, and all the other factory-produced ingredients that cascade down the nutrition "facts" on labels. This is the nutrient stream that has made its way into the system that produces foods for all of us and, unfortunately, for the next generation as well. It is a result of a fast-paced, fast-food society that has relinquished the power of food choice and quality to government regulations and corporate bottom lines.

"Healthy" food is not exempt from this travesty. There are plenty of healthy junk foods on the market as well. Foods that are labeled "natural" and "whole" can still contain ingredients that are completely processed. Other labeling terms are merely misleading. "Fat-free," for example, means that the product has less than half a gram of fat, not that the product contains zero fat.[3] "Low fat," "low carb," "low sodium," and "low in sugar" can also be misleading. Even the foods that are labeled "fresh," "lean," or "extra lean," such as meat, may not be as healthy or beneficial as implied. Take a package of ground beef as an example. The beef is advertised as 80 to 90 percent lean. This means that there is 10 to 20 percent fat still in the ground beef. Pork, beef, and other supermarket meats can be labeled "lean" if they are no more than 10 percent fat and "extra lean" if they are no more than 5 percent.[4] Depending on the weight of the package, it could potentially add up to quite a lot of hidden fat.

"Fresh" is also a vague term, and it does not always mean "good for you." If you live in the Northeast and you buy "fresh" raspberries in

February, you can be assured that they were not picked locally that day. Most likely they have come from somewhere outside the country, sprayed with chemicals to prevent decay and pests, packaged, placed in a crate, shipped to an airport, flown to a regional distributor, packed on the back of a truck, driven to your market, and then, eventually, after at least one week and up to three, find themselves ready for sale in your supermarket. Remember, the longer a berry, fruit, or vegetable takes to get from a plant, the earth, or a tree to you, the more nutrients it has lost along the way.

The freshness of fish is similar, especially any that come from large commercial fishing boats. These boats leave the dock and go out for up to two weeks before they return with their catch. During the voyage, the fish are packed in storage containers of heavily salted ice-cold water or tons of ice. By the time the fish gets to your plate, you might add on another week, maybe more. Yet this process is still labeled "fresh."

There are also labels that tell us that the product inside the box or jar is "enriched" or "fortified" with one type of nutrient, vitamin, or fiber. Do not think that you are getting double the nutrients here. *Fortified* products have nutrients added to them that were not present in their whole state. *Enriched* products are those that have undergone some type of processing that removed all of their beneficial properties, so the manufacturers have had to add these nutrients back in. This process is most common in flours, boxed cereals, and pastas and is part of the federal guidelines and state mandates given to manufacturers as a result of the nutrient-deficient diets and the processed foods that Americans and people in many other countries thrive on.[5] Interestingly, these guidelines are not enough to force these manufacturers to include the nutrients that they removed without actually being mandated to do so. As Ronald Schmidt and Gary Rodrick point out in their *Food Safety Handbook*, "contrary to popular belief enrichment of grain products is not a federal mandate. States are free to enact their own laws or policies regarding the availability of enriched products. Federal authority lies only in the standards of identity for enriched products."[6] As an example of how food manufacturers are more concerned with the bottom line than with your health, take a look at the debate on folic acid fortification in the United Kingdom. Folic acid, or folate, has been shown to prevent birth defects, but it is removed during the refinement of grains. The British government encouraged processors to add it back in, but with limited success. As the *Journal of Chemistry and Industry* reported, an industry representative explained that the failure to comply with the government's mandate was because "nobody is going to get rich off of this. It's not a new blockbuster drug that's going to bring in $200bn. Nobody makes money off of this except the healthcare system."[7]

Ultimately, what all these labels and containers and packaging amount to is garbage—not just for our bodies, but also for the environment. Whether it is plastics, papers, Styrofoam, or disposable diapers, these products have become a very large part of our municipal waste stream. The great Pacific Garbage Patch stretches from the coast of California to the coast of Japan and contains an estimated 3.5 million tons of garbage, according to the United Nations Environment Program, 90 percent of which is said to be land-based sources such as plastic from food containers, shopping bags, and water bottles that overtake sea life by a ratio of 6:1.[8] The United States is fortunate to have an established system of waste management and recycling, but many other countries do not. Elsewhere around the world, plastic and other food packaging are openly burned. Not only does this create major toxicity and respiratory problems on a local level, but it adds to the global currents of air and water as well as makes the land upon which it is burned toxic.

Think about and monitor your own garbage. How much of it is packaging, and how much of that packaging is related to your food consumption? The garbage that you see on your local beaches, streets, and woods is a direct result of the purchases and product choices we make every day. The closer you bring yourself to your community—where the option of buying non-packaged products at farm stands or green grocers is easily possible—the more you will see the impact that this type of nonbiodegradable packaging waste has on the environment.

The one thing you can be sure of is that the farther you get from a food's source and the more packaging a food has, the more processing it has undergone and the more nutrients it has lost from its original state. Anything that can be bought in a can, jar, box, or container

is not a pure, whole food. Pick an apple from a tree and eat it; that's a whole food. Pick the same apple, freeze it for a year or process it into a frozen pie or jarred sauce, and it is no longer the same fruit. Once a food begins to undergo a transformation from its natural form, it starts to lose its nutrient value. Apples, for instance, help lower cholesterol, are a mild antibacterial and anti-inflammatory, are high in fiber, and can help suppress the appetite. All of these properties become diminished or lost in processing. Maintaining the majority of your vegetables in their raw state for consumption is the best way to retain their nutritional properties.

When you do need to purchase grocery items such as grains, pastas, nuts, seeds, and even dried spices, doing so from the bulk section of your supermarket or natural foods store is the best way to go. You can eliminate the packaging that you would normally bring home and discard by shopping with your own bags or containers (I have some Ziplocs that are over five years old!). Buying grains, pasta, and the like in bulk also ensures that you are not going to eat unwanted preservatives.

Eat What You Need—Follow Your Instincts

Active lifestyles require food; how much is always a question. There are formulas you can use to calculate your daily caloric intake, and I have included some of these formulas in the "Sports Nutrition" chapter. Note, however, that they are rough guidelines at best. Dr. John

Ivy, a doctor who developed one of the formulas, noted in conversation that "their purpose is really just as a guide."[9] Trying to calculate food intake relative to a daily caloric value is something that works better in a laboratory than in an athlete's kitchen. It's far better for active athletes to follow their instincts on how much to eat. To do so successfully, however, you must first base your diet on whole foods, for it is only when your body is getting the nutrients it needs that you can then use your intuition to fulfill your athletic requirements.

It is also important to understand and acknowledge that not all nutritious natural foods are available to us at all times and in all places. Learning to store and cook many of these non-seasonal foods will allow us to keep, say, tomatoes on hand in the dead of winter in Maine.

The habits of wild animals serve as examples of using intuition to stay healthy and active. Animals are, in essence, the original athletes, often traveling long distances, climbing, running, and swimming, while always on the lookout for foods that support these efforts and their subsequent survival. In his book *Racing the Antelope*, Bernd Heinrich gives an example of the pronghorn antelope having a "perfect running physique. It eats the right kinds of vegetation without knowing anything about diet. It simply obeys its hungers and aversions, selecting food from the diverse menu it encounters in its environment."[10]

Using our food instincts, instead of counting calories or adapting unreasonable quick-fix diets, is something basic yet essential. For gold medal Olympic speed skater Apollo Anton

Ohno, his instincts are his best nutritional asset. When asked about his daily caloric intake, he said, "It all depends on my activity level. I've never really counted calories because when I'm in tune with my nutrition, I can feel when I need to add more grams of fat, protein, or carbohydrates."[11] As Ohno has discovered, activity level is a highly individual matter. Do not base your food intake on someone else's routine. Learn to support your body with the foods available to you, in the quantities you need, prepared in the time that you have.

Overeating can be a problem for a lot of athletes. As a result of frequent exercise, an athlete's metabolism is active, dynamic, and demanding. However, exercise is not an excuse for indulgence in just any high-caloric foods; high-quality whole foods are critical for the body's ability to absorb nutrients and satisfy the body's demands without overeating and weight gain. Metabolism is a two-part process. Most people are familiar with the digestive part of metabolism, known as catabolism. This is the process where the body breaks down food for its nutrients and extracts the energy it needs for its daily functions and activities. Once food is broken down, the nutrients are absorbed into the bloodstream and then distributed throughout the body's cells. It is a system that was designed for whole foods. Processed foods are hard for the body to digest because they do not contain the necessary digestive enzymes that whole foods do, particularly natural foods that are raw. Consequently, processed foods become a calorie load rather than a high-quality source of energy. Your body continues to eat more food in search of the nutrients that it needs, and that food becomes unwanted weight.

The other part of metabolism is known as anabolism. This is the buildup process that occurs within the body for the creation of muscle proteins from amino acids. Here again, the quality of one's food is essential to the ability of the body to function effectively. Or, to say it more simply: what you put into your body will determine what you get out of your body, and the food you use to build your body will determine the strength of the structure of that body.

How does this translate into an eating strategy? For those of us whose schedules are somewhat unpredictable and filled with travel, work, or raising children, eating smaller meals in addition to snacks throughout the day is the most successful approach to maintaining a healthy metabolism. This approach provides you with the opportunity to properly time your food intake in relation to your training schedule without running into the issue of overeating. Those with more predictable days and routine training times can eat fewer snacks and slightly larger meals that fulfill your nutrient requirements. Individuals who are not necessarily training but are still physically active need to choose the approach that works best for them.

A good place to start is with a small meal of somewhere between 300 and 500 calories, possibly more, depending on your total caloric goal for the day. The recipes in this book, including the fresh juices and snacks, are perfect to use as you begin this simple process.

A handful of mixed nuts and a piece of fruit, whole-grain bread with nut butter spread and banana, or a small salad with some seeds and nuts can all be considered for your small meal.

Eating smaller meals throughout the day (approximately every two hours) allows you to keep your body consistently fueled while your metabolism is simultaneously breaking down those foods to provide the nutrients necessary to produce the energy you need to support your athletic activities. You can also adjust the size of your meals to master your time schedule, breaking the day into shorter meal times instead of worrying about providing yourself with those nutrients at the usual three opportunities a day that longer meals entail.

Don't Let Yourself Get Hungry

Becoming hungry is one of the most common nutritional pitfalls that plague people with busy schedules and active lifestyles. And doing so can be the nutritional breaking point of one's entire day. There is a difference between your mind telling you that you are hungry and your body telling you that you are hungry. Thankfully, the difference is generally pretty easy to distinguish. Physical hunger is the point at which you begin to feel your blood sugar drop, you start to lose focus on the task that is in front of you, and your stomach feels empty and begins to grumble. These all are signs that your engine is running low on fuel. The next phase of this is a feeling most everyone has experienced: the fight-or-flight mode, where food of any kind becomes an easy solution. In a society that has access to literally thousands of choices of convenience foods, hunger is a situation that is easy to resolve.

For those who are nutritionally unprepared, the answer to hunger pains is convenience snacks—foods that are easy to grab and, unfortunately, highly processed with refined carbohydrates, sugars, and fats, and totally not what your body needs. They are the snack foods available in office vending machines, the fried whatever from the corner deli, or those tasty chips, candy, and other junk foods that are easily accessible and calling out to you. These foods provide satiety for the body because of the quick uptake of sugars and the fullness within the digestive system. These are also the foods that send your body on those sugar highs and lows, the ones that rank high on the glycemic index. Once you start down this path, the body starts to crave them and the mind generally gives in. You can't let this happen. It is at this point that a trained mind and body work together. Your mind will have learned, based on the nutritious foods you have been feeding it, that you do not want to take that food direction, that when you want to call upon your body to exercise and train, these junk foods can inhibit any benefit you might have derived from your workout.

The only time you should be hungry is when you wake up in the morning. This signifies that your eating habits the day before were spot-on. Your last meal should come at least two hours before you go to bed and should not be the typical large dinner that most Americans consume. The energy requirements of the body before bedtime are minimal and only need to support the most basic metabolic tasks. Even if you have a late training session, your timing for food recovery should be such that dinner does not need to be a lot of food. When you awake in the morning, your body should be ready for you to start up your metabolic engine. Once you stoke the fire of your metabolism with breakfast, it is important to keep that flame on a steady burn throughout the day. However, it is not necessary to fill yourself up every time you eat; by the time you reach "full," you will most likely have overeaten. Try to eat until you feel almost full, and be sure to drink enough water with your food. If you give your body time to begin digesting what you have already eaten before getting to the point of feeling full, you will see that you can be satiated with less than you thought.

Small meals throughout the day tend to satisfy an athlete's eating requirements because the body's response to hunger generally begins around two hours after the last food intake. Topping off the body every few hours keeps it supplied with the nutrients it needs, stabilizes blood sugar, and prepares it to absorb the fuel it needs to support your athletic endeavors.

Preparation Is the Answer

Preparation is to cooking as training is to racing. Successful execution of virtually anything we do requires planning and preparation. To make nutrition part of your lifestyle, you need to prepare in advance to successfully carry out the plan.

Preparing whole foods gives us the opportunity to understand our connection to the earth and appreciate the offerings cultivated from the soil by local farmers. The excuse I most often hear for not cooking is a lack of time. But if we do not allow time in our lives to prepare the best meals for our bodies, we relinquish our food choices and food quality to an agribusiness that developed one-stop shopping as a solution for busy schedules. If, however, we embrace the cycles of the earth, time management will become very easy.

As a private chef, I am often asked by my clients what I am going to prepare. My usual answer, which some find troubling at first, is, "I don't know; I need to see what they have at the farm stand before I can create a menu." Though this method might raise worries and seem unorganized, you will soon find that you can actually save time and reduce stress when you prepare your meals according to seasonally available foods. The act of cooking begins not when your food hits the pan but when you purchase the meal's ingredients.

Preparation is the only solution to never allowing yourself to get hungry and has many options. Access to healthy food can always be possible when properly managed. Give yourself the time to research and prepare wholesome snacks in advance. Stock your workplace with easy-to-store foods such as dried fruit, nuts, seeds, popcorn, a small jar of nut or coconut butter, and cured olives. In your fridge have hummus, sprouted tortillas, fresh salsa, jars of kimchi or pickles, and other items that are easy to eat and don't have to be frequently replenished due to spoilage. You can also have some components like a salad dressing, tapenade, dulse, or miso paste that can be used to "healthy up" things like store-bought salad greens, roasted chicken, or a sandwich a colleague picked up for you.

Never Cook One Meal at a Time

Of course, one of the joys of a delicious meal is its leftovers. When it comes time to prepare the ingredients for a meal, my suggestion is to never cook just that one meal. Instead, think ahead. You can add fresh foods to leftover ingredients as the week goes on or take them along to your workplace or training venue.

As you can see, if you are really committed to having a solid nutrition plan, you need to spend time in the kitchen. Setting two to three hours aside once a week to prepare meals and snacks for the days to come will go a long way toward allowing you to eat well and save time later. Prepping and cooking can also be a nice way of capping off your day or getting ready for the week ahead, as well as a way to keep your body moving while cooling down after training. Doing so with your family is a great opportunity to spend time together and, for your children, to instill a solid foundation about food. Inviting a training partner or friend over to help cook also makes for a fun experience and shares the workload.

Here is how one of these evenings might unfold after your trip to the market. Start with a whole chicken, which you can roast in the oven or on top of the stove. Roasted chicken is a great center point for cooking and can be used in a variety of ways for other meals. It is also a great family meal, and you can easily roast more than one at a time. The chicken requires just over an hour of active cooking and about 15 minutes to allow it to rest. Now that you are already in the kitchen, you might as well take advantage of the time there. If you planned in advance, you would have soaked some grains and beans the night before. Even before you start the chicken, you can cook the beans as well as some grains. If you haven't planned that far ahead, start soaking them for the next day. If you are soaking quinoa, remember it takes the same amount of time to cook two cups of quinoa as it does one, so make enough for the next few meals.

Fill the sink with water and rinse the veggies you just bought at the farmers' market— kale and broccoli, for example. Shake off the excess water, tear off the kale leaves, and set them aside. Cut the broccoli into florets. A few minutes before the quinoa is ready, you can add some broccoli to a bamboo steamer and place it on top to cook.

Now go through the rest of the things you bought. There may be some peppers that you want to cut up for burritos. Are there herbs

you want to put in some water? Are there bush beans that need to be trimmed? The idea is to take advantage of the time you have and put it to work for you.

Preparation is nothing more than thinking ahead to use your time to your advantage. For example, never let boiling water be used for just one purpose. You can always make use of the steam to cook vegetables, or you can strain the water over some vegetables for a quick blanch. Same goes for the oven: while roasting the chicken it can also cook root vegetables such as beets, yams, or heirloom potatoes, enough for that night's dinner and for snacks and meals to follow.

When the quinoa is done, you can use some immediately for a salad to which you can add some of the kale. Set the rest aside to cool and finish off the next day. By the time the chicken is done, you have not only dinner for that evening but prepared foods and ingredients to be used for the rest of the week. With the oven off, place apples or peaches inside to take advantage of the residual heat so the fruit is just warm enough to be used as a dessert. A little planning, good humor, and practice will have you on your way.

During the week when you are preparing meals, your preparation beforehand continues to be instrumental to your success, not only for the quality of your food but also as a time-saving mechanism. In fact, preparation is so important that in the culinary world the French phrase *mise en place* is used to describe it; it essentially means getting your ingredients together before you start cooking. As you do this, think further ahead. Doubling your recipes takes no more time to prepare and leaves you with leftovers for another day.

Keep Your Pantry and Fridge Well Stocked

Having a well-stocked pantry and fridge with ingredients that enhance fresh foods is essential in preparing nutritious balanced meals and saving time. You can use the list in the "Resources" chapter as a guide and add your own favorites to it. Once you have this continually revolving arsenal of components established, cooking becomes easy and creative. Turn leftover quinoa into a salad with some cured olives, sprouted pumpkin seeds, and fresh herbs. Add to that a bit of roasted chicken and you've prepared dinner in less than 10 minutes. If you have made any of the spreads in the "Recipes" chapter, put the spread and some veggies on sprouted tortillas and have a quick sandwich in even less time. Or simply pick up an apple or a pear while you are out to turn your nut butter or tahini into a great snack. The more ingredients you have in your pantry, the easier it will be to create quick nutritious meals. It is a dynamic process that will keep you involved with your own food preparation, keep your palate excited, and never leave you hungry or nutritionally depleted.

4

General Nutrition

Whether you are an Ironman athlete with a training schedule of 20 hours per week, a regular gym attendee, or simply someone who enjoys the outdoors, making the right nutritional choices is essential to living a healthy and active lifestyle. When you are dedicated to nutritious eating, it becomes a basic part of your life. The knowledge, practice, and dedication you have to keeping your body healthy make it easier to make the right food choices. While some of the decisions you have made will become an ingrained part of your daily routine, following through on these decisions requires practicing a few regular mental check-ins.

Choosing foods that are healthy, fresh, and organic may, at first, be an overwhelming adjustment if you have been shopping in traditional supermarkets that lack these choices. But cooking with and eating fresh, wholesome foods that contain the basic nutrients our bodies need to allow us to be active and healthy—including fats, calories, and carbohydrates—have never been more important. As the previous chapters have made clear, our food supply has become convoluted and depleted—so much so that the Food and Drug Administration found it necessary to release a set of guidelines for manufacturers explaining what a whole grain actually is, which foods qualify, and how they should be labeled.[1]

Also, in response to the degradation of our food supply, a number of organizations have been started to raise awareness and act as watchdogs over the food industry. One of these organizations is the Whole Grains

Council, which provides consumer education on whole grains, sponsors research, and serves as a liaison among science, industry, and consumers. (See Chapter 7, "Resources," for information on other watchdog organizations.)

People always ask me whether organic foods are really better for you. An industry with $24.6 billion worth of sales in 2008 and that has experienced annual growth of almost 20 percent over the past decade is clearly not just a passing fad, and there's a reason for this.[2] Organic foods address some basic issues of food safety and nutrition; more to the point, though, is that studies have shown that organic produce has up to 50 percent more nutrient value, depending on the item, than conventional produce.[3] And this concentrated nutrient value is exactly what athletes and active individuals need to sustain their energy requirements.

If you are an athlete, you put quality time into your training and getting your body prepared for the demands you ask of it. It's the only vehicle you have for performance. Don't you think it deserves the best fuel and food you can buy? The same question can be asked of those who don't consider themselves athletes but are simply trying to get the most out of life. Our daily nutrition is the platform on which all of life's activities are built. For most of you, it might require looking in a different direction—such as a farmers' market—to find the foods that will support your lifestyle. The additional expense may seem an issue at first, but when your food has twice the amount of nutrients, the overall cost will be lower in the long run.

The bright golden "Whole Grain" stamps that appear on packages containing legitimate whole-grain products consistently identify three levels of whole grains in a serving. A "Good Source" has 8 grams (half a Dietary Guidelines serving), an "Excellent Source" has 16 grams (a full Dietary Guidelines serving), and a "100 percent Excellent Source" (also a full whole-grain serving) has all its grain content as whole grains.

For those of us interested in optimal health, making the right choices in our diet is crucial. With the dizzying array of foods that line the aisles of our supermarkets, arming yourself with as much nutritional information as possible is imperative for making the best selections. Eating natural unprocessed foods that are low in additives and preservatives but high in energy value can add diversity to your diet while increasing the nutrient content of every meal. You can also experience the joy of eating more often, having more energy, being prepared for your fitness requirements, and reaching your athletic goals.

Know the Difference Between Supplements and Enhancements

I have a bittersweet relationship with technology and innovation. I love the technology in carbon-fiber equipment, green surfboards, lightweight climbing Camalots, and aerodynamic bicycles as much as anyone. But when it comes to food and diets, I tend to think that technology, in the form of supplements, is more of a harmful bandage placed on nutrient-deficient food and improper eating than an asset to health and athletic performance. To supplement or not to supplement remains a question often asked by athletes and individuals trying to maintain a healthy diet and obtain an extra performance edge. However, there is no substitute for a diet based on whole foods; there are only enhancements.

The packaged foods that constitute much of the common daily diet do not supply the essential nutrients that our bodies need. As a result, athletes and active individuals looking for a quick fix are often driven to buy pills that are allegedly filled with the nutrition that an active body requires. But vitamin pills and supplements will not provide the nutrients that raw, natural foods will.

The demand for vitamins and food supplements has made the vitamin industry a multi-billion-dollar business. Ironically enough, this has occurred, at least in part, for the same reason that the organic food industry has flourished: people are looking for a better source of complete nutrition. So-called nutrition centers and vitamin shops have erupted across America's landscape, each of them containing dozens of sections that look as if they are stocked with leftovers from Halloween (and a look at the ingredients shows that the majority of them are equally as scary). The problem with this approach is that people do not understand that nutrition and what they eat—what they put into their bodies—build a holistic organism. Instead, the search for one particular

nutrient, isolated into a supplemental form to provide a performance boost or immune protection, becomes a patch on poor overall nutrition. As the popularity of these supplements shifts and becomes debunked over time, the one constant that emerges is the knowledge of harm relative to nutrient deficiency rather than the supplementation thereof. Unfortunately, many professional athletes, trainers, and individuals also do not possess the requisite knowledge about the effects of these supplements or how they work in the body, yet they still choose to use them. As a result, one of the most disheartening issues at stake today is that young athletes see nutritional supplementation as the primary key to performance enhancement.

The nutrients contained in tablets and capsules exist in isolation, but, says Dr. Thomas Cowan, author of *The Fourfold Path to Healing*, "Our bodies were not meant to take isolated nutrients."[4] When found in food, vitamins have many counterparts that assist the body in absorption and digestion. Isolating these nutrients in high doses is a process your body would never be subject to, even if you were eating the healthiest diet possible. Nutrients work with others not only from the same foods but also from vitamins, minerals, and fats that can be found in other whole foods. These compounds activate each other to make them soluble for the body's metabolism. When nutrients, vitamins, and minerals are not working in concert with their counterparts or are without the active enzymes to digest them, the body will be unable to absorb them fully for maximum benefit. Whole foods in their natural state are the best source of nutrients. There is simply no argument. Vitamins as supplements are nothing more than that.

Common supplements that I am often asked about, specifically for athletes, are branched-chain amino acids, creatine phosphate, glucosamine and chondroitin, caffeine, and vitamin C. I will discuss these in the next chapter on sports nutrition, but the point I would like to make here is that the effects of supplements on performance are limited in their scope, and when isolated from their natural sources they have the same issues as any other processed vitamin. To concentrate on one secret or magic item that is going to optimize your performance is a misguided approach. Relying on a bottle of pills for your nutrient supply as a supplementation to whole foods is a hard road to travel. If you want the security of knowing that you are ready to step up to the starting line, then you must focus on your overall dietary consumption.

Instead of taking supplements, a better idea would be to consider "enhancements." These are whole food sources and products that support an already established diet of natural, seasonally fresh, and traditional foods. There are a number of nutrients that the body cannot produce on its own, and the only way to get them is from the earth's bounty. Because athletes have busy lifestyles, some nutrients can be convenient to consume in a simple nonsupplementary format, without the availability of the entire food itself. One of these key nutrients is essential fatty acids, particularly found in fermented cod liver, hempseed oil, and flax-

seed oil. Another whole food source I recommend for athletes on the go is my own product, SunPower Greens, which is a comprehensive source of vitamins, minerals, and probiotics. Both of these enhancements are healthy additions to a regular diet based on the high-quality foods that lead to sustainable success.

Food as Fuel: Energy Bars and Drinks

It is important to understand that food as fuel and food as a means to address hunger are two different concepts. Packaged energy foods and drinks are "fuel foods" specifically designed as a convenient fuel supply for athletes who are training or racing over a period of time at high intensity. They should not become substitutes for real food nutrients needed throughout the day. Energy foods, whether bars, gels, or drinks, are concentrated to be high in calories and carbohydrates. Most of them, though, are low in nutrients. Their purpose is not to satisfy your hunger while you are working at your desk or driving your car, or as a substitute for whole foods, but to fuel your exercise requirements. Liz Applegate, PhD, author of *Encyclopedia of Sports and Fitness Nutrition*, cautions people "not to replace whole foods with energy bars" and suggests that "energy bars are for anyone who is exercising 1 hour or more, after which they need an external source of carbohydrates."[5]

Eating these products instead of real natural foods at any time of the day except during a workout does nothing but load you up on extra calories that you do not need. The food industry has capitalized on the concept of "healthy fast food," and many companies have created what they call "food bars." For the most part, these are simply processed products similar to all other packaged foods, with a mix of ingredients that may or may not come from good sources. Some are better than others, with a higher nutrient quality, particularly those that are raw. But even the better-for-you food bars should be limited to a minimal portion of your diet. Leave them for the times when you truly need them—before, during, or after a strenuous workout—and restrict your consumption of the gels and drinks to long training sessions and races. At all other times, strive to eat real food, prepared at home with the best ingredients you can find. See the recipes in this book for healthy suggestions that will fill your nutritional needs without supplements.

Weight Loss and Weight Gain

Simply put, the number of overweight and obese people in the United States is totally out of control. In fact, obesity has become such a worldwide problem that it's earned its own moniker: "globesity."[6] According to the World Health Organization, in 2005 there were 1.6 billion people considered to be obese and 400 million people considered to be overweight.[7] U.S. statistics for obese men and women were over 33 and 35 percent, respectively, in 2005–2006,[8] and the Centers for Disease Control reports that from 2003 to 2006 the prevalence of obesity in children was 17 percent in ages 6–11, and 17.6 percent in ages 12–19.[9] The definition of *obesity* is an accumulation of excess body fat that frequently results in significant and life-threatening health issues, with the body fat calculated through measurement of one's body mass index (BMI), which is based on the relationship between weight and height.

I think it is important to note that such statistics did not exist 50 years ago. The effects that processed foods have had on the overall health of people in the United States—and now throughout the Western world—and the tendency for many of them to be overweight slowly took time to register in the education, science, and health fields.

Even active people who do pay attention to their food intake can struggle with weight issues. Athletes in particular focus on calories, not wanting to take in too many for fear of carrying around extra weight and thereby losing strength, power, and/or endurance. The problem with this preoccupation is that the focus is on calories and not nutrition. Calories are a source of energy, but for optimum health and physical performance calories need to be derived from whole nutrients, not from the empty calories found in processed carbohydrates and the like. When considering calories, it is important to remember that, like food, they can be split into two basic groups: the calories needed while training (fuel) and those needed for sustenance to carry you through the rest of the day (food). Food calories are needed to maintain energy levels for work, social activities, and, most important, to provide the foundation for one's fueling program while exercising. They are also the critical components that our bodies use for repair and replenishment after working out, and are the calories that we need to be concerned about for weight gain and loss. "Fueling calories" are defined as those specific to meet the needs and efforts of your training session or workout; I will look closely at them in the next chapter.

Whether you've made a recent resolution to exercise more; are gearing up for a marathon, triathlon, or other competition; or are just trying to shed a few pounds, weight loss—like anything that has to do with nutrition—is person-specific. No two people lose weight in the same way. The method you use to control or lose weight is determined by your goals, motivation, body type, metabolism, schedule, and commitment. For those who want to achieve their ideal weight, a simple reduction in portion size at each meal will do the trick. But for anyone with poor nutritional habits, weight control requires more than just dietary modifications. In addition to overhauling what you eat, your routine will need to be accompanied by an increase in physical activity. In other words, eat less, eat better, and move more! Create a calorie deficit, whereby you burn more calories than you consume.

To keep the weight off, you need to incorporate a dynamic, sustainable routine that is easy to modify using your own instincts—which, by now, should be based on whole foods, as opposed to following a "diet" that someone else has created for a broad population and not specifically for you. Formulaic diet routines that take a shotgun approach to weight control tend to create more problems for individuals that fall outside the diet's narrow parameters, and most of them therefore wind up being short-lived experiences.

Remember, too, that it is natural for an athlete's weight to fluctuate over the course of a year based on training requirements, the race schedule, injuries, and the general flow of the seasons. Do not overreact to these fluctuations. To sustain a natural rhythm, eat what you need, not what you want, and focus on creating nutritionally complete meals that supply your body with a variety of whole foods. You will find that although your weight may rise and fall through the year, it will not swing wildly in either direction, and you will naturally find the body weight that is most comfortable for your health.

For some, there may be times when gaining weight is necessary to support one's athletic endeavors. Gaining weight can be accomplished by slowly increasing one's food intake to match the increase in training intensities and subsequent requirements. To achieve weight gain (or loss), I have experimented with various formulas based on counting calories, carbs, fats, and so forth, but none has ever succeeded. The only successful approach I have found, for others and for myself, is to maintain a nutrient-dense diet while continuing to follow a regular exercise program. This is a model that is sustainable.

Daily Caloric Requirements

Being in tune with your body and allowing yourself to make necessary changes take time. Determining your ideal weight by the numbers on a scale or through clothes size is potentially harmful. A focus on nutrition is primordial, and my system will help you maintain that focus for the rest of your life. But getting there can be an understandable challenge for some, and in these cases, calculating caloric intake or expenditure can be helpful, especially for those who do not trust their eating instincts or who have not yet developed good habits. These formulas do not replace a holistic approach to one's nutrition and should always be used with the understanding that they will not produce precise answers, only general indications.

The first step in understanding your daily caloric requirement is to determine your total daily energy expenditure (TDEE). This is the total number of calories (energy) that your body needs while taking into account all of your daily activities. There are two calculations that will get you closest to the general vicinity of your needs: the Harris-Benedict equation, which is based on total body weight, and the Katch-McArdle formula, which is based on lean body weight. Both of these formulas will provide your basal metabolic rate (BMR) first, which measures the amount of calories necessary to support your basic bodily functions and organs while at rest. This is a more comprehensive approach than using the general factors of height, weight, sex, and age that other formulas employ. With your BMR in hand, you can then use an "activity multiplier" to reflect your level of activity, which in turn will determine your TDEE.

The Katch-McArdle formula is the more complicated and specific of the two, in that it requires a measurement of your body composition along with a subsequent calculation of your lean body mass. Your doctor may be able to perform the measurement, or you may be able to get it at a sports medicine facility or sports clinic. You can then use the lean body mass number in the formula to determine your BMR. An example of the Katch-McArdle formula, for men and women, is:

$$BMR = 370 + (21.6 \times \text{lean body mass in kilograms})$$

The Harris-Benedict formula is simpler because it uses only total body weight:

$$\text{Women: } BMR = 655 + (4.35 \times \text{weight in pounds}) +$$
$$(4.7 \times \text{height in inches}) - (4.7 \times \text{age})$$

$$\text{Men: } BMR = 66 + (6.23 \times \text{weight in pounds}) +$$
$$(12.7 \times \text{height in inches}) - (6.8 \times \text{age})$$

Once you have your BMR from either of these formulas, you can use the activity multiplier to determine your TDEE:

$$\text{Sedentary} = BMR \times 1.2 \text{ (little or no exercise, desk job)}$$

$$\text{Lightly active} = BMR \times 1.375 \text{ (light exercise/sports}$$
$$\text{1 to 3 days per week)}$$

Moderately active = BMR x 1.55 (moderate exercise/sports
3 to 5 days per week)

Very active = BMR x 1.725 (hard exercise/sports
6 to 7 days per week)

Extra active = BMR x 1.9 (hard daily exercise/sports
and physical job or twice-a-day training, i.e.,
marathon, triathlon, professional game, etc.)

There are also many online calculators available that simplify the measurement process. None of them is likely to be as accurate as either of the preceding formulas, but they are quick and easy to use. The Mayo Clinic's online calorie calculator is a good starting point; go to www.mayoclinic.com and type "calorie calculator" in the search box. Once you have determined your optimal daily caloric intake, you will need to calculate the caloric values of the foods you eat based on their portion size, which in turn will require weighing your meal portions on a food scale and calculating total calories. These methods of counting calories for weight loss or weight gain are beyond the scope of this book, but there are many online calorie calculators that can simplify the process.

More Is Less

One of the best methods I have found to control hunger spikes, moderate cravings, eat less, add more diversity to my diet, and control my weight is to increase the frequency of my meals but decrease the portion size. In other words, I never let myself get hungry. Most people, including athletes, eat two or three big meals a day, dinner being the biggest, with unhealthy snacks in between. As a result their metabolism is never in sync with their body or supporting its needs. This traditional eating schedule can lead to hunger pangs, fatigue, impulsively eating foods that are high in fat, becoming overweight with related health issues, and getting next to no nutrition. Changing this routine to allow for three smaller meals per day with two or three healthy snacks in between can help control these issues.

One fact to keep in mind is that fats can be good for you if they are of the healthy varieties that come from organically grown vegetables, fruits, nuts, and pasture-raised animals. Fats are a necessary component of a healthy diet and will add to your satiety, aid the absorption of fat-soluble nutrients, and help stoke the carbohydrate flame. Cutting fats tends to be a cornerstone of many weight-loss programs and diets, but the body needs fat for optimal health. Most people on a low-fat diet wind up eating an abundance of processed foods that are completely devoid of nutrients and do not take into account the body's needs. The no- or low-fat programs lead to major food cravings, loss of energy, poor digestion, and a host of other issues. It is an approach that I have never seen work for long-term success, and I believe it is especially incompatible with an athletic or active lifestyle.

Break the Fast

The term *breakfast* literally means "to break the fast," and it's a term everyone should take very much to heart. One of the most overused, outdated, and dangerous tactics that people incorporate when trying to lose weight is skipping breakfast. Although calories play a role in losing weight, it is the quality of those calories that is most important. Simply eliminating them may get you to your short-term goal a bit faster, but without any accompanying lifestyle modifications this approach will not serve you in the long run. By skipping meals, especially breakfast, you are depriving your body of essential nutrients that it needs to perform not only the basic functions of your day but also those that require a bit more energy for exercise. Breakfast provides the body with nourishment after its overnight fast and the energy it needs before a morning workout. Skipping breakfast only continues the night's lack of food and may hinder your ability to put forth the effort in training required to achieve your fitness and racing goals.

Equally important, but often overlooked, is the fact that eating breakfast jump-starts your metabolism for the day. In doing so, your body will immediately begin to consume and use calories for energy. By keeping that metabolism at a slow burn throughout the day with smaller meals, your body will constantly be consuming calories—provided they are the ones that are nutrient-dense with live enzymes to allow for proper digestion. Foods containing medium-chain triglycerides like coconut oil will also help increase the basal temperature of the body and subsequently the metabolism, thereby helping one lose weight as well. If you watch animals in the wild or at pasture, you will see them grazing almost all day long, especially during winter. This action is what stimulates heat production in their bodies, keeping them warm and lean. The engine is always running. Athletes can benefit from the same approach, starting the day with a good breakfast and then "grazing" throughout the day on healthy food, while avoiding overloading the body with three heavy meals.

In the end, skipping meals is a signal to the body that it needs to retain as many calories as possible. As a result, these calories ultimately end up in the body being stored as fat instead of being used for work, muscle building, and repair. A recent study published in the *American Journal of Epidemiology* found that skipping breakfast was linked with a greater chance of obesity. People who skipped breakfast were more than four times more likely to be obese than those who ate breakfast daily.[10]

Start Big and End Small

Most people choose to eat their biggest meal at the end of the day, after the body has completed its exercise-related energy requirements, allowing all of those calories to just sit around. Some of these calories will be used for replenishment and energy, but the majority will be cast aside and stored as fat. By doing the opposite and eating the bigger meal at the beginning of the day, you will provide your body with the necessary fueling for all of its energy requirements and not leave a surplus at the end. Knowing what to eat is only part of the challenge of nutrition; knowing *when* to eat is the other part. By putting these two parts together into a fitness program, you will have a formula for success.

The Programless Program

What all of this essentially amounts to is a program without a program. I have never seen a dietary intake—a "diet"—laid out in such a way that it could possibly encompass all the people who attempt to use it, with all of their different energy requirements and varying physical characteristics. In fact, I have yet to see a "diet" or "program" that works in a sustainable fashion. It is true that most people undertaking diets see early results because they are making a modification to their lifestyle that their bodies must accommodate. But I rarely see a useful, long-term improvement from these diets. In fact, at my clients' urging I have prepared meals from an array of what I refer to as "fashion diets," the ones that come and go in their faddish fashion, and what I have found is that they lack flexibility, food quality, and a supportive lifestyle.

The guidelines and concepts in this book are a reflection of nature because nature is a dynamic process. It has the ability to adapt to changes. We all change through the differing seasons of our lives, and subsequently so do our nutritional requirements. This occurs not only over the course of a lifetime but also within a year, a month, and even a week. Trying to incorporate a regimen that does not have the ability to reflect these changes can lead to isolation, questions about what to do next, and, worst of all, a situation that sets one up for failure. As a result, returning to old habits becomes a potential reduction of self-image and an indulgence in improper foods, both of which continue to play off each other until one attempts the next latest and greatest diet. Strict diet programs do not change as you do. They remain the same no matter what you bring to them, and I have never seen anything succeed in the long term based on that approach. What I have created is the framework for a sustainable program that you can change as often as you need to, as long as you adhere to and maintain the core principles.

Where do you go when your fashion diet does not address a situation in your lifestyle? A telephone support line with a flowchart of the book you already have? A box of products, powders, and supplements that your body is beginning to reject? At what point will you be able to rely on yourself for the answers when your kitchen is filled with fresh, beautiful whole foods that you can feel good about? The guidelines and recipes within this book will give you the tools to mold your changing dietary requirements for as long as you live, with a system that will never let you down. Using the credos will provide you with all of the answers you could ever need to help you make the right choices for yourself.

What I find equally imperative is to understand that your diet is not just about you. Your food choices are directly related to the health of your local environment, and ultimately the health of the world. It is irresponsible to expect that the earth should support you if you do not take the time to care for it. That would be a completely unsustainable concept and one that places the individual alone at the center of the universe. However, each of us is only passing through the place called earth. The choices you make about how you eat are a reflection of the way you choose to live while you are here and how you want to leave the planet once you are gone. The quality of the food choices you make will ultimately determine the health of your local environment, and you will most certainly be one of the many benefactors.

5

Sports Nutrition

Nutrition is the most overlooked essential element in an athlete's lifestyle, which is ironic given that disregard for nutrition can negate every effort put forth in training and competition. Because the physical demands of sports go beyond the daily requirements of the body and its natural resilience, the absence of a balanced diet that incorporates this understanding can lead to grave consequences, such as injury and illness.

Exercise, athletics, and recreational sports are supposed to be fun, but implementing the science of sports nutrition into a daily routine can prove to be a great challenge. For most, the normal response to the first sight of nutritional formulas is a sprint straight to the cookie jar! Even some of the world's top professional athletes, when left to their own devices, do not know how to make proper nutritional choices and fail to follow a holistic approach to eating, training, and maintaining the health of their bodies. Instead, they end up eating easily accessible "sports foods" or highly processed "fast" foods.

The most important thing to understand is that *your athletic nutrition plan is only as good as your everyday nutrition plan*. Having a solid base on which to build is crucial for everyone who wishes to participate in any fitness- or sports-related endeavor. A lifestyle of proper eating and nutrition is important to aid in the recovery and repair of stressed muscles; replenish the body with nutrients; allow the body to take advantage of increased fitness, strength, and stamina; and provide a platform for your body's energy and nutrient requirements. This knowledge and understanding is part of the holistic package described in the previous chapters of this book. If any of its parts are neglected or ignored, the rest of that package will be affected as well.

As you saw in the previous chapter, no one vitamin or nutrient is more important than any other; all must be kept in balance. Now that you understand how the nutrients that come from whole foods are based on how we take care of those food resources and the earth, determining your athletic nutritional and caloric requirements is the next step. Whether you are training for an Ironman distance triathlon, surfing on weekends, or competing in recreational sports, you are going to have to do some minor calculations if you want your nutritional intake to support those endeavors and your athletic goals.

A sports nutrition diet can be broken down into three stages of when, what, and how much to eat in pre-training, during training, and post-training. The post-training period is the most important stage, as it blends in with your daily nutrition routine and plays a critical role in recovery. All of these stages will be discussed in detail in this chapter.

Sports scientists agree that the "aerobic diet" should be composed of approximately 55 to 70 percent carbohydrates, 25 to 35 percent fats, and 10 to 15 percent proteins. Depending on your stage of training and the intensity and duration of the workout or event, these numbers will vary somewhat, but as you can see, carbohydrates lead the pack of macronutrients. What people fear most in their diet is what you get to indulge in. So, call your friends and tell them to bring over those whole grains and running shoes!

This diet is the universal template for juniors and adults, including triathletes (long- or short-course), runners, cyclists, climbers, surfers, swimmers, and anyone who participates in aerobic activities on a regular basis. Your new-found holistic intuition is still going to be your best source of information to tailor your personal requirements, but you can also use some simple calculations to give yourself guidelines to work within. These numbers are based on your daily caloric requirements, which can be calculated using the formula for your basal metabolic rate (BMR), your sports/exercise caloric requirements (which are based on the intensity and duration of your training), and your weight. Basal metabolic rate was discussed in the previous chapter; the other formulas will be discussed later in this chapter.

This chapter will help you understand the specifics of sports nutrition. The holistic concepts and organic foods that you incorporate into your lifestyle do not change. There are also some "sports fueling products," or sports foods, that are better for you than others. But, again, these are no substitute for whole natural foods. When you have developed into a high-performance athletic machine by using the best-quality ingredients, the last thing you want to do is derail that machine with inferior fuel.

The Aerobic Diet

Essentially, the aerobic diet is one that sustains an efficient relationship among the macronutrients (carbohydrates, fats, and proteins) that support the body's energy requirements and its ability to train with intensity and endurance. However, adenosine triphosphate (ATP) is the only source of energy that can drive muscle contraction.[1] As your energy requirements increase from simple workouts to endurance training, so too does the requirement for ATP. It is produced in the body in three different ways, two of which are anaerobic and one that is aerobic. These processes are driven by the supply of stored nutrients—creatine phosphate and glycogen via glycolysis for the anaerobic system, and macronutrients for the aerobic system—via cellular respiration. Endurance athletes primarily use the aerobic system for sustained fitness routines (hence the importance of the aerobic diet). They also rely on the anaerobic process for higher-intensity efforts, such as running up steep hills or bursts of speed that require immediate energy. However, both aerobic and anaerobic processes work together over the course of an event or workout.

The body's primary source of energy is the aerobic system, which can burn carbohydrates, fats, and proteins, and the efficiency of this system relies on the body's ability to deliver oxygen to the working muscles during maximum output, a state known as VO_2max. When our energy requirements increase such that the body cannot deliver oxygen fast enough to produce ATP, it adds the anaerobic system as a supplemental energy source, where carbohydrates become the only fuel source through a process called anaerobic glycolysis. The drawback to glycolysis is that it can last for only a few minutes, at which point it produces a product called lactate faster than it can be processed into energy. The result is the muscle burn that every athlete is familiar with, and which serves as a warning for the body to back off and allow it to return to the aerobic system for its energy source. As the aerobic engine takes over, the lactate continues to be processed, thereby allowing the anaerobic system to be ready for another higher-intensity "push." The greater the intensity of the exercise, the more carbohydrates contribute as a source of fuel.

In the general population, most people eat way too many carbohydrates, but for athletes they are the body's preferred source of fuel for aerobic activity. To be very clear, the aerobic diet is solely for the use of athletes and individuals who are working out at high intensities for durations of at least 75 minutes once or twice a day, and five to six times per week. For everyone else—those living active lifestyles, working out 45 to 60 minutes per day, five days a week, where the exercise is something like yoga or taking short runs—the basic whole foods diet described in previous chapters is entirely adequate. Here's why.

During digestion, the body breaks down carbohydrates into glucose and then transports it through the circulatory system on a preferential basis to the muscles and then finally into the liver, where it is stored for later use. This stored glucose is what we know as glycogen and is essentially the body's storage form of carbohydrate. Glycogen that is stored in the liver is released into the bloodstream to maintain adequate blood sugar levels, whereas glycogen that is stored in the muscles can be seen as a reservoir that the working muscles draw upon as needed. During exercise, the stored glycogen is converted back to glucose, at which point it is available to be used for energy. Individuals who are working out for less than 60 minutes have enough stored glycogen to support their efforts. There are approximately 300 to 500 grams of stored carbohydrate in the muscles, which is equivalent to about 1,200 to 2,000 calories' worth of energy (each gram of carbohydrate yields roughly 4 calories). Prolonged exercise requires initial levels of glycogen storage banks to be topped off in order to sustain the effort because as the work intensity increases, carbohydrate utilization also increases. This will be discussed further under "Fueling for the Competition."

Fats and proteins are also used for the production of ATP as a source of energy through the aerobic process, but neither is as efficient as carbohydrates. The overuse of protein can lead to muscle breakdown, as well as the by-product ammonia, which is harmful to the kidneys and muscles. Fats do not break down fast enough in the body to support energy needs. Moreover, fats require the presence of carbohydrates to be used as energy—hence the expression "fat burns in a carbohydrate flame."

If you maintain your glycogen stores, your body will become more adept at using them for your energy requirements. With adequate glycogen stores onboard, protein will contribute only around 5 percent of the energy needed for ATP production. However, when glycogen stores are low, that number could reach 15 percent, which can cause dehydration and an inefficient fuel source, which points to the importance of maintaining rich sources of carbohydrate in your daily meals.

Nevertheless, fats and proteins are very important in our overall diet. Fats promote the absorption of fat-soluble nutrients that are critical in supporting the athletic body, and are a source of omega-3 fatty acids. Proteins and their building blocks, amino acids, are essential for numerous bodily functions that range from repair and recovery of muscles, organs, and ligaments to helping deliver carbohydrates to particular parts of the body.

Determining how to achieve a nutritional balance is easier when you are in tune with your body and its requirements. Author and professor Bernd Heinrich's path to the ultramarathoners' Hall of Fame came about through experimenting constantly with his nutrition and allowing his body to guide him. Although food choices vary among athletes, the aerobic diet has proven its worth. The Tarahumara Indians of northern Mexico are probably the world's greatest running culture, where, for some, running over 50 miles per day is the norm and up to 75 percent of their diet is complex carbohydrates. The Kenyan runners of the Kalenjin tribe, whose competitive running is unsurpassed, maintain a regular consumption of food that very closely resembles the aerobic diet.

The aerobic diet is for overall daily consumption and can be generally determined using the BMR formulas described below. As a general rule one should consume at least 45 calories per kilogram of body weight per day if training a minimum of 1.5 hours per day overall. To get a number in the range of 60 percent carbohydrates, multiply your weight in pounds by 3.2 for lesser intensities and by 4 for higher intensities. Or, in general, athletes should consume 9 to 10 grams of carbohydrate per kilogram of body weight (or approximately 36 to 40 calories), 1 to 2 grams of protein per kilogram of body weight (4 to 8 calories), and 1 gram of fat per kilogram of body weight (9 calories) per day. (To figure body weight in kilograms, multiply pounds by 2.2.) Those who are active and not in rigorous training can cut these numbers in half. Keep in mind that these are just general guidelines and need to be adjusted to each individual and his or her particular needs.

Understanding Macronutrients and Micronutrients

Carbohydrates

Carbohydrates, the first of the three big macronutrients, come in two forms: simple and complex. Simple carbohydrates, also known as simple sugars, are generally found in candy and sweets (table sugar, chewing gum, soft drinks) and are also present in fruits (apples, cherries, oranges). Not all simple sugars need to be avoided, especially those found in fruits, but they should be consumed at proper times to be beneficial. In sports food products you will see them listed in processed forms, such as sucrose from beets or cane, glucose from grape juice, fructose from fruits, maltose from grains, and lactose from milk. Still, your best source for these sugars is unrefined whole foods. Morning is a good time to incorporate some simple sugars into your diet because they will help jump-start your body's metabolism as well as replenish liver glycogen that your body used while sleeping. Post-exercise is another good time for simple sugars so that the body can quickly uptake and replenish glycogen stores.

Overall, however, athletes should focus on eating complex carbohydrates. They can be found in whole grains, cereals and pastas such as whole wheat, spelt or rye bread, brown rice, quinoa, oatmeal, beans, and root vegetables. These foods should be the main source of complex carbohydrates in an athlete's diet. Typically, sports food products contain complex carbohydrates in the form of maltodextrin, which generally comes from GMO corn, potatoes, or rice, unless otherwise specified, and glucose polymers (due to their slower release time). In addition, complex carbohydrates contain necessary B vitamins that the body needs to effectively use the carbohydrate and provide a source that will be slowly released into the bloodstream. This will give your body the sustained energy requirements for a long-distance competitive event, as opposed to the quick high and low that simple carbohydrates provide.

An understanding of the glycemic index (GI) can also help you make judicious choices about which carbohydrates you choose to consume as well as when to consume them. The GI was created to help diabetics rank the speed with which a food affects blood glucose levels—or, to put it another way, how quickly a food is likely to raise blood sugar and insulin levels. Interestingly, the numbers are not always what you might expect; for example, you might assume that ice cream, a simple carbohydrate, would affect the bloodstream more rapidly than a bagel, but the opposite is true. As Denise Feeley, an adjunct professor of nutrition and athletic counselor at George Washington University, told me in an interview, "Not all foods act in the body the way we might think they should."

The GI ranks foods according to a scale: The higher the food ranks on the scale, the quicker the sugars enter the bloodstream. High-glycemic foods have an index greater than 70, moderate-glycemic foods between 55 and 70, and low-glycemic foods less than 55. You can find various iterations of the GI scale online.

Although we can divide carbohydrates into defined molecular groups, each body reacts to and processes them differently. In addition, food synergy plays a role in the effect of carbohydrates on blood sugar. The rate at which carbohydrates enter the blood is determined in part by the amount of dietary fiber, the type of fiber, the fat, and the protein contained in the food as well as the foods that are being eaten

with it. As I have already stressed, the athlete's main focus should be on incorporating a diversity of fresh, whole foods into the diet and balancing that intake to meet the body's requirements and demands. Doing so will relieve you from reliance upon the GI. The recipes in this book represent that balanced approach to eating, and the book also includes specific recommendations in the pre-workout, workout, and post-workout sections later in this chapter. The GI alone will not provide you with a winning edge, but an understanding of how it works can play a role in your nutrition action plan. Ultimately, a comprehensive approach to nutrition is the best recipe for confidence at the starting line.

Fats

Contrary to popular belief, fats play an important role in the diet of an athlete. Specifically, essential fatty acids (EFAs), which the body cannot produce, are required for the production of eicosanoids, which regulate blood pressure, blood viscosity, vasoconstriction, and immune response.[2] Fats also play an important role in the production and maintenance of healthy cells. Saturated fat provides stiffness or integrity to the cell wall, and cholesterol makes it waterproof.[3] Without saturated fat and cholesterol, the cell wall cannot transfer beneficial nutrients and waste properly. In addition, cholesterol is a precursor to vitamin D as well as the steroid hormones estrogen and testosterone.

Plenty of athletes maintain a low-fat diet thinking that it will increase lean muscle mass.

However, some studies have shown that a low-fat diet can lead to a decrease in athletic performance in addition to compromised health.[4] Trained athletes have been shown to be excellent fat burners, and fats have over twice as much caloric energy per gram (1 gram of fat packs 9 calories) as carbohydrates and proteins. As a result, fats can be an excellent energy source for extended exercise. In fact, fats are best used to fuel exercise of low to moderate intensity, or up to 65 percent of VO_2max, after which carbohydrates become the predominant source of fuel. The majority of fats consumed are triglycerides and are stored in the adipose tissue of the body, which is the surface layer beneath the skin. In sports food products, medium-chain triglycerides (MCTs) are often used because they go directly to the liver for storage and are much more readily available. Coconut and palm oil, mentioned earlier for their beneficial role in raising basal metabolic rates, are good food sources of MCTs for athletes.

Proteins

The third source of energy for aerobic ATP production is protein. Most athletes imagine their protein needs to be well above their actual requirements, and protein's benefits for athletes have yet to be fully researched and established. Part of the overconsumption of protein has to do with its availability, but for athletes in rigorous training it is also part of the body's natural mechanism to gravitate toward the foods that it needs. (This is another reason why being in tune with one's body is one of the most critical parts to a successful nutritional program. I know for myself that when I experimented with specific numeric guidelines, I felt suboptimal and saw a negative effect in my training. When I shifted my dietary habits to meet the needs of my body, I noticed an immediate difference in not only my athletic performance but also my overall physical and emotional constitution.)

An easy guideline to keep in mind for your overall diet is that endurance athletes can consume approximately 0.7 to 1.2 grams of protein per pound of body weight per day. For added strength and muscle building, a bit more than that is appropriate, while for subendurance pursuits it can be a bit less. Proteins are composed of amino acids. There are twenty-two standard amino acids, of which eight are known as "essential" because the body cannot produce them; they must be obtained from foods we eat. Some foods, such as fish, eggs, cheese, and meat, are known as complete proteins because they contain all of the essential amino acids in adequate proportions. Quinoa, buckwheat, amaranth, soybeans, hemp seeds, spirulina, and Aphanizomenon flos-aquae (AFA, a type of algae) are also complete proteins. There are also complementary foods, such as beans and rice and hummus (a blend of chickpeas and sesame seeds), that create complete proteins. Plants (grains, legumes, and vegetables) can be excellent sources of some proteins, but most are incomplete and should be combined with other foods. This is another example why having a diversified whole foods diet is so important to daily health.

In sports food products that are heavily processed, protein is generally listed as whey protein or soy protein concentrate or isolate, or hydrolyzed or textured soy protein. Soy protein isolate begins with defatted soybean meal and then goes through a number of caustic and hazardous chemical washes before it becomes the final product. The majority of soybeans grown in this country are also GMOs. Whey protein can be a better choice if it comes from a good source and has been processed with care, but most whey is a by-product of the industrial dairy manufacturing process of making cheese and comes from those animals I described earlier, the ones pumped with hormones and pharmaceuticals and given GMO feed. The other important concern with whey or soy protein is its overconsumption and concentration. Soy products are commonly used in recovery drinks, and it can be very easy to consume much more than is necessary, potentially resulting in damage to the kidneys and liver, where proteins are broken down. Too much processed soy can also cause digestive stress and other gastrointestinal issues. Many athletes don't like to eat immediately after working out, which makes these products popular because they are easy to consume. But you can easily prepare your own recovery drinks using better-quality whole foods. Easy alternatives, such as a smoothie made with yogurt or raw milk, hemp seeds or hemp powder, SunPower Greens, or nut butter with an apple or sprouted bread, will provide you with proper nutrition. If you do choose to use a recovery product with protein for convenience sake,

try to purchase one made with organic whole foods from non-GMO sources.

Proteins rank third behind carbohydrates and fats as an energy source, even though they have the same amount of calories per gram as carbohydrates. The main role of amino acids in proteins is to build and repair new tissues and muscles, hormones, enzymes, and antibodies. Proteins also are responsible for the transportation of nutrients and blood balancing and are an integral part of the immune system. Only for endurance events do proteins become more of a contributor to energy needs, where they can add up to 15 percent of the total energy used. As noted earlier, however, protein usage at this rate is not desirable, and maintaining adequate glycogen storage is imperative to keep protein usage below this percentage. Training—specifically endurance training—helps the athlete better utilize proteins as well as glycogen.

Micronutrients

Macronutrients tend to get all the attention in any discussion of nutrition, and as a result micronutrients can become a forgotten or neglected part of the equation. They are only "micro" in their direct relationship to energy production and the small amounts that are necessary for the body. But micronutrients such as iron, iodine, calcium, chloride, and magnesium, as well as vitamins A, C, D, E, K and the B vitamins, play a very major role in daily nutrition. Without them the body would neither be able to fully utilize the macronutrients nor be able to produce enzymes, hormones, and other substances necessary for proper growth and development and be healthy enough to perform physical activity.[5] Vitamins and minerals are especially important for athletes in the daily diet because they help maintain the systems necessary for training and recovery.

As important as micronutrients are, trying to monitor their daily intake to maintain them in specific quantities is an almost insurmountable task. Fortunately, it is also unnecessary if you maintain a natural whole foods diet. If you follow the credos in this book and use the recommended methods of cooking and the recipes, you can maintain the micronutrients your body needs, realize the health benefits of a balanced diet, and optimize your athletic performance without any additional effort. This is what organic performance is all about.

Sports Supplements vs. Enhancements

In a world of increasing competition, athletes are constantly looking for the latest and greatest item to help them get to the finish line first or faster. Having the best new equipment, however, can rarely be kept a secret. As a result, sport-specific nutritional supplements have joined the list of hoped-for secret-in-a-bottle gear for many athletes. They are generally affordable, especially as compared to new equipment, and can also be kept and used somewhat clandestinely as the information slowly trickles through the sporting community. Whether they actually work or not, most every athlete is at least willing to try them once or twice.

Even for sport-specific purposes, though, supplements are best viewed as enhancements to a well-established whole foods diet. There are a few that can add some benefit to an athlete's health due to the additional stress placed on his or her body as well as help to aid in athletic performance. But with enough diligence and attention paid to one's diet, there is generally no need for processed supplements.

Ergogenic (energy-generating) aids are beneficial primarily to endurance athletes while training and competing. The most common ergogenic aid is caffeine. Its benefits are also controversial. Studies by Terry Graham, PhD, and Lawrence Spriet, PhD, professors of human biology and nutritional sciences at the University of Guelph in Ontario, Canada, have produced results that support caffeine as a beneficial aid in athletic performance. These studies indicate that caffeine is effective for events of low intensity and endurance, like trail running and long-course triathlons, as opposed to events that require high intensity, like climbing, surfing, and sprinting.[6] The beneficial role that caffeine plays is explained by Dan Benardot, an associate professor in the Department of Nutrition at Georgia State University, who says, "caffeine assists in the mobilization of free fatty acids, that are stored in the muscles, into cells where they can then be metabolized."[7] Studies have shown that this action delays the immediate depletion of glycogen during the first 15 minutes of exercise, reducing its loss by 50 percent.[8] As a result, the saved glycogen can be used later in the workout when it would not normally be available. Keep in mind that this has not proven to be an ongoing benefit after those first 15 minutes have passed.

Other studies suggest that cause for the delay in fatigue has to do more with an athlete's perception of effort and an increase of mental alertness. There is no guarantee that either of these benefits will work for everyone. In addition, as with anything that has an upside, there is a downside. This is certainly the case with caffeine. Possible side effects of caffeine include sleep deprivation, nausea, cramping, fatigue, headaches, anxiety, gastrointestinal distress, and dehydration. Again, it is important to remember that these side effects vary from person to person. If caffeine in coffee does not sit well with you, use green tea instead (and benefit from its additional antioxidant properties as well).

Dehydration is a major concern for athletes who use caffeine, as it is a mild diuretic. Caffeine increases the blood flow to the kidneys and inhibits the reabsorption of sodium and water. Tolerance is also an issue to consider. Those who consume caffeine on a daily basis will find it has a lesser effect as a beneficial aid. Removing caffeine from your diet at least seven days prior to an event will help offset this. Be mindful as well about the source of caffeine that is contained in sports food products. Natural sources are always the best, and over-the-counter products that contain caffeine can be very hard on your body's system.

One supplement that is generally unknown to most athlètes but that can benefit endurance and aerobic activities is Coenzyme Q10 (CoQ10). It is referred to as an ubiquinone because it is a naturally occurring enzyme that is found everywhere in the body, though it is mostly concentrated within the heart. It is beneficial to athletes in its ATP production and for its antioxidant properties. However, these benefits have not been widely researched within the scientific community, and there are questions as to whether these enzymes have beneficial effects for healthy individuals. As a result, there are no specific dosage suggestions.

Vitamin C is another ubiquitously found element in the body. It serves many functions; as an antioxidant, vitamin C helps eliminate free radicals created by oxidative stress and also helps boost the immune system. For athletes this is important due to the increased levels of cortisol released in the body and due to physical stress that can lead to sickness. Vitamin C also helps with the absorption of iron, which is beneficial to hemoglobin and red blood cells and, subsequently, oxygen that is carried throughout the body. There are many food sources of vitamin C, such as strawberries, watermelon, mango, oranges, lemons, raw sauerkraut and other lacto-fermented foods, leafy greens, broccoli, asparagus, tomatoes, and sweet potatoes. In supplemental form vitamin C can be known as ascorbic acid, and it is very often a GMO by-product. When making my own sports drinks I will sometimes add pure acerola powder, because it is a whole food source of vitamin C that does not contain any potentially harmful ingredients.

Branched-chain amino acids (BCAAs), glucosamine and chondroitin, and creatine phosphate are a few other commonly used supplements worth mentioning due to their popularity. BCAAs such as valine, leucine, and isoleucine are found in many foods and are considered essential for their energy synthesis. Most amino acids are processed in the liver, but BCAAs are metabolized directly in the muscles via a special synthesis that can be enhanced during exercise. Supplements with BCAAs taken before exercise may have the same effect. Note, however, that any specific benefits for increased performance are unproven. Given their unique ability to build muscle as well as stop the breakdown, I find them to be an important part of my recovery foods. Maintaining a well-balanced diet will provide your body with plenty of BCAAs.

Creatine phosphate is part of the anaerobic process of ATP production used during high-intensity workouts. Its use is beneficial for muscle and strength building, which is why it is commonly found in products targeted for those sports. There is no scientific evidence to support its use for endurance or aerobic activities or as a supplement to be taken while exercising.

Glucosamine and chondroitin have been widely studied and promoted to athletes who experience injuries from overuse of muscles and stress on certain joints. It is believed that they prevent the breakdown of joint cartilage or promote the growth of cartilage and provide relief from joint pain. Both of these compounds are readily manufactured in the body, so their intake and advantage are predicated on the "more is better" philosophy. Although

the effects of glucosamine and chondroitin have been studied, the studies have focused on the compounds individually and not when they are taken together, so any claimed synergistic benefits are unproven. Many people take them as a preventive measure, but no studies have been done on the efficacy of their use for this purpose. However, I can say from personal experience that taking glucosamine and chondroitin has helped with the maintenance and recovery of joint injuries. In supplements they are sourced from shellfish and animal cartilage. Most studies claim that there are no foods that contain both glucosamine and chondroitin, but you can get chondroitin into your diet by eating the cartilage around the joints of chicken bones.[9]

The quest continues to find that leading edge for athletes, but a proper and well-balanced diet allows your body to maintain itself in the way that keeps you healthy and active. What the body doesn't produce from within, nature will provide in the whole foods that you eat. The most important thing to understand about sports food products is that all of the sources of their ingredients—unless they are organic—are generally made from highly processed GMOs. They can be convenient for the athlete but can also have negative effects on the body and environment that may or may not be immediately apparent. Your best bet as an athlete is to focus on your daily nutrition and support that with a nutritional strategy based on timing of intake and quality of foods. Without a solid foundation to start with, it does not matter how many supplements you take; your performance will never benefit from them.

Timing Is Everything

The human body and its biological functions operate correctly based on physiology and the input of proper nutrients. The demands placed upon the body for physical training and competition create an additional set of circumstances that can greatly increase the body's abilities to perform and recover. The proper ongoing management of this cycle is the most important realization an athlete makes, secondary to the quality of nutrients he or she enjoys. Correct management will add to the prevention of trauma-related injuries and dehydration, will aid in recuperation, and will provide a source of continuous fuel to accomplish the challenges athletes face.

There are three stages of physical activity that require precise nutritional management: before, during, and after the activity. However, individual success lies in the ability to view them holistically as part of an overall plan tied into one's daily nutrition. The degree of participation and diligence—paying attention to your own needs and creating a plan that fulfills these needs—is the key to longevity in any sport. It is an ongoing process. There is no one plan that can be exactly replicated for everyone. An athlete never shows up for an event with the exact same body and weather conditions. Complete success in any sport requires thought and action based on the needs your body may have experienced in previous situations and your subsequent ability to foresee them as a result of proper training and eating.

Pre-Training Nutrition

Adequate fuel consumption prior to exercising for sessions lasting beyond 60 minutes is a crucial requirement in order for you to meet the energy and physical demands of the rigors and stress your body undergoes. The goals at this stage are to boost blood glucose, top off liver glycogen, spare the use of muscle glycogen, and help stall the increase of cortisol in the body, which will break down enzymes and create illness. Maintaining a diet based on a diversity of whole grains, fruits, vegetables, healthy fats, fish, and meats is the first step. Understanding your personal requirements relative to the duration and intensity of your session is the second step. The third is to ensure that your fuel source is devoid of simple refined sugars, has a good source of complex carbohydrates, meets the quality that your body and environment deserve, and is something that you enjoy. Timing is the piece that completes the puzzle. What you eat, what form you consume it in, and how much are all predicated on personal timing. As with all nutrition components, there are some basic guidelines and strategies that are important to understand and that can be adjusted specifically to your body and your routine. What works for one does not necessarily work for all; only through experimenting will you find the answers that work for you.

First and foremost, it is important to recognize that for the body to adequately use the fuel provided before a workout, it needs to be in an optimally "recovered" state. Viewing nutrition holistically will provide you with the perspective to understand that pre-training fueling actually begins with post-training replenishment. For those of you who are training with twice-a-day, back-to-back, or extra-long workouts, this should be your mantra. Trying to fuel an already depleted body will only perpetuate a deficient cycle that will ultimately lead to its breakdown.

There is no dispute that eating prior to workouts improves training. It's a pretty simple concept; you don't expect your car to get very far without fuel, and neither will you. But the quantity of fuel you choose is something that is individually specific. When you choose to train is dependent on the personal factors of your life, such as work and family, and it is important to identify those elements and understand how they will affect your ability to properly fuel and hydrate prior to exercising. You should also consider your digestive ability or stomach tolerance, because that can play a big role in determining your nutritional plan, fuel choice, and timing.

There are two distinct metabolic periods that guide the timing of food/fuel consumption. The first is approximately three hours before working out or training, and the second is 30 to 60 minutes prior to training. Professional athletes tend to follow this routine naturally, but everyone should do so if they can, which will impart the flexibility to time fueling consumption without running into the issue of overeating, gastrointestinal distress, or insuffi-

cient amounts of fuel. Research indicates that fueling (that is, eating) during each of these metabolic periods improves performance during training.

Ideally, the pre-training meal takes place three hours prior to the beginning of a workout. Studies have determined that complex carbs are the body's first choice for endurance energy. They are easy for the body to digest and provide a sustained source of energy. Pre-training fuel intake, therefore, should be composed of 65 to 70 percent carbohydrates. A good guideline for most individuals who work out is between 200 and 400 total calories, with 0.5 to 1.0 gram of carbohydrate per kilogram of body weight. Consuming this meal three hours ahead will allow the body enough digestive time to assimilate the nutrients and glycogen and empty the stomach of its contents. This also gives the body enough time to regain its hormonal balance after any blood sugar and insulin response it may have had. In addition, by consuming enough complex carbs and allowing enough time for digestion after eating, your body can use carbs as fuel at the onset of exercise as opposed to using fats or proteins. If your body is particularly sensitive to having a spike in blood sugar, timing your meals around three hours before training and consuming complex carbs are even more important.

Simple carbohydrates or sugars by themselves are not recommended because they can create a negative glycemic response or hypoglycemia (low blood sugar) as a result of the body's need to release insulin to carry those sugars into the blood. Initially the body will feel a quick high, but this will then be followed by a crash once those sugars are used. There is no doubt that this type of situation can and will impede performance. Try to avoid sports foods or fueling products such as energy bars that use only simple sugars, like fructose and sucrose, as a source of carbs. Although they are convenient and taste good, they do not provide a sustainable source of energy. If you prefer these bars for convenience, try to find ones that have at least a mix of both high- and low-glycemic carbs; the low carbs will slow the release of the high carbs.

Cooked whole grains like quinoa, which is also a great source of branched-chain amino acids; grains that are sprouted and used for breads, such as spelt, barley, and rye; and brown rice are great choices as pre-training foods. Legumes are also good sources of complex carbs, but avoid those that are high in fiber as they are more difficult to digest and typically create gastrointestinal distress. High-fiber carbs may also create a need for an unplanned bathroom stop during your session.

Many athletes can be very superstitious and want to eat the same thing before every event, game, or training session. This is fine if you compete on a fairly infrequent basis, so long as the meal meets the necessary nutrient requirements. Eating the same meal on a nightly or daily basis, however, is not a good idea. The monotony of the same foods will not provide the quality and diversity of nutrients that the body needs on an ongoing basis.

Proteins and unhealthy fats should be kept toward the lower range of the aerobic diet for pre-training fuel. According to Dr. John Ivy from the University of Texas, a carbs-to-protein ratio of 4:1 has proven to work very well on tested athletes by improving their endurance during exercise.[10] Protein is important, as it helps carry the carbs into the muscles, helps to reduce muscle damage during exercise, and is also a minor source of energy for the body. However, too much protein will delay gastric emptying time and will create gastrointestinal distress as a result.

Any pre-training meal based on whole foods should also include some healthy fats. These fats, which are extremely important to a well-planned diet, come from oils found in flax seed and hemp seed; from cold-water fish like mackerel, bluefish, and tuna; and from avocados, coconuts, and tree nuts. Fats help satisfy hunger, but too much and the wrong kind will cause trouble. Avoid those fats that are "trans" and hydrogenated. These will slow down the digestive system and inhibit the body's ability to increase its heart rate. They are also poor sources of primary fuel for endurance athletes. The body does use fats as an energy source to "fuel the carbohydrate flame," but high fat ingestion will hamper the body's ability to do this.

Sometimes, eating just one to two hours prior to training is a must for busy athletes. If you have an early morning session, your body has used some of its stored fuel during the night and requires replenishment. (See "Fueling for the Competition" for some strategies for morning food consumption for an event.) Consume the most easily digestible forms of carbs and other foods possible. Smoothies are a good option, as are simple foods like yogurt and granola, hummus, or miso soup with soba noodles. Portion control is a crucial component at this time. If you are going to be eating two hours prior to training at moderate intensity, a good guideline is to consume around 0.5 gram of carbs per pound of body weight. For example, a 135-pound female would consume approximately 68 grams of carbohydrates. This could be done with one or two slices of sprouted whole-grain bread topped with a small bit of nut or seed butter and agave nectar.

Note that some studies suggest that eating less than three hours prior to exercising can lead to a faster rate of depletion of muscle glycogen. These studies recommend that athletes wait until 5 to 10 minutes prior to beginning exercise and consume 100 to 200 easily digestible calories at this time. My own experience does not support this approach, but if you find that eating two to three hours prior to training is not providing sufficient fuel, you can experiment with this recommendation.

Thirty to sixty minutes before training is the time period when the actual fueling begins. Rather than think about food, focus on consuming fluids and some nutrients that can really benefit your performance. This is the time to top off your glycogen stores, blood glucose, and insulin levels. If your stomach has an empty feeling and you are hungry around an hour prior to training, a couple of bites of something simple tend to do the trick. I will have a macaroon, a couple of dates, or dried pineapple and some water just to appease my hunger, avoiding anything heavier than that.

Eating solid foods 30 minutes before training is for those whose stomachs can properly handle it. For some, it would be better to drink a sports drink with electrolytes. Coconut water is a good option because it allows you to hydrate at the same time you are taking in nutrients. There is no specific guideline for the amount of liquid you should consume, but 12 to 20 ounces is a good ballpark figure. You do not want to drink so much that you will feel bloated; you just want enough to get you going. The addition of electrolytes will help your body retain and properly use the fluids.

Getting to a training session on a daily basis can be difficult in itself, and being under-fueled only makes it harder; in addition, it can lead to a successive breakdown later in the day. The most important thing is to time your larger meal so that by the time you are within 30 minutes of starting your training, you are just adding essential nutrients to what is already there. Although the body is compared to an engine metaphorically, it is not one in reality and cannot take advantage of filling its tank just before it needs the fuel. Doing so will only cause distress to the digestive system, along with potential dehydration due to the water that is needed to aid in the process. Although the overall nutritional concept is to be looked at holistically, how your body responds to the demands of training is more closely related to how well it is fueled.

Nutrition During Training

The second stage of sports nutrition is the time you spend training, and it is the time to practice

TABLE 5.1: ENERGY EXPENDITURE VALUES

Activity	Energy Expenditure Value (cal/min/lb)	Activity	Energy Expenditure Value (cal/min/lb)
Aerobics: high-impact	.07	Running: 5.5 min/mile	.10
Aerobics: low-impact	.04	Running: 6 min/mile	.13
Basketball	.06	Running: 7 min/mile	.11
Cycling: 10 mph	.06	Running: 8 min/mile	.09
Cycling: 15 mph	.08	Running: 9 min/mile	.09
Cycling: 17.5 mph	.09	Running: 11.5 min/mile	.06
Cycling: > 20 mph	.12	Ski racing	.06
Football	.07	Soccer (competitive)	.08
Hockey	.06	Strength training: circuit	.06
Ice climbing	.06	Strength training: vigorous	.05
Kayaking	.06	Surfing	.05
Mountain biking	.06	Swimming backstroke	.08
Mountaineering	.04	Swimming breaststroke	.07
Paddleboard surfing	.06–.07	Swimming freestyle: 50 yards/min	.06
Rock climbing	.05	Swimming freestyle: 75 yards/min	.08
Running, cross-country	.07	Tennis match	.08

Source: Adapted from J. Ivy and R. Portman, *The Performance Zone: Your Nutrition Action Plan for Greater Endurance & Sports Performance* (Laguna Beach, CA: Basic Health, 2004), 61. Reprinted by permission of Basic Health Publications, Inc., and J. Ivy.

and refine your race-day fueling plan. It is during this stage that the trial and error of all your experimenting is realized. This includes the experimenting you've done during your pre- and post-training stages. Everything you've learned about your nutrition is aimed at the results you achieve while training and competing. Athletes are constantly experimenting with different fueling techniques to understand the best methods for their success. The supplement industry relies on it. Ultimately, the goal of nutrition and an aerobic diet practiced during training and competition is to delay fatigue for as long as possible. Given that exercising is a calorie-deficit process—because the body cannot absorb and replace equal amounts of calories burned or ounces of fluid lost—fueling during these times becomes an effort to replace as much as the body can take and rely on the storage of glycogen, protein, and free fatty acids for the rest. In doing so, you are also aiming to prevent dehydration and electrolyte loss, reduce muscle damage, bolster the immune system, and provide a foundation for post-exercise consumption that will aid in faster recovery and repair of the body.

The aerobic diet is aimed at the overall daily food consumption of an athlete. The time spent actually exercising, training, or competing has its own set of caloric requirements, which vary for each individual. Even then, the requirements for any one individual change depending on a variety of factors. In general, caloric requirements are based on the intensity and duration of exercise and the weight of the individual. Additionally, personal fitness, temperature and humidity, stress, types of food and fuel used, dietary regime, thermoregulation, timing of intake, and the possibility of unknowns all contribute to how a body processes its caloric needs. Having a range to work with helps while creating your race- or event-day nutritional intake, but it is crucial for the athlete to establish that range well before that day comes.

The best calculation of the range of one's caloric needs I have found is described by Drs. John Ivy and Robert Portman in their book *The Performance Zone*. The first step is to determine your total calories burned for an entire exercise session using the following formula (see Table 5.1 for the energy expenditure values):

(body weight in pounds) x (length of session in minutes) x
(the metabolic equivalent of the session intensity)

For example, a 150-pound person exercising for 120 minutes at an intensity of 0.1 (for example, running a 7-minute mile) equals 1,800 total calories. Multiply that by 0.25 and you get 450, which is divided in half to get the amount of total calories needed per hour, 225. The concept of replacing each calorie burned with an equal calorie consumed is one that will lead to disaster. The body cannot absorb equivalent calories during exercise, so the goal should be to consume about 25 percent of the total calories used.

To determine the breakdown of nutrients, multiply 225 by between 0.55 and 0.75 (55 to 75 percent) for carbohydrates, 0.10 to 0.15 (10 to 15 percent) for proteins, and 0.25 and 0.35 (25 to 35 percent) for fats; this will give you the calories needed for each session. To convert the calories to grams, divide carbohydrates and proteins by 4 and fats by 9. Use Table 5.1, adapted from *The Performance Zone* by Ivy and Portman, for metabolic equivalents.

The most important number here is the one you determine for carbohydrates. In the example above, 225 calories per hour yields a range of 146 to 169 carbohydrate calories, or 37 to 42 grams.

Another formula, suggested by Dan Benardot, is simply to consume 1 gram of carbohydrate per minute of exercise. This formula does not take into account body size or intensity, and may or may not allow you to maintain adequate glycogen stores in your body. However, given that the maximum amount of carbohydrates that the body can absorb during an hour is 50 to 70 grams, this formula provides a very easy place to begin. Another formula you can try, very similar to Benardot's, is 1 gram carbohydrate per kilogram of body weight per hour. Hence, a 154-pound person would consume 70 grams of carbohydrate per hour, or 280 calories. This is the upper level at which most bodies can convert carbs to glycogen. An amount above that can potentially cause gastrointestinal distress.

There are also online sites that allow you to log your exercise regime and create daily food logs that will help you track your caloric requirements. Because these sites are static, they should be used solely as starting-point guidelines. Many variables come into play over the course of training that can affect dietary intake. Regardless of the formula you choose, make sure to test it thoroughly and in a variety of training situations before using it as a lead-in to your big competition.

Although carbohydrates are king when it comes to fueling your body, they cannot do it alone. As I mentioned earlier, up to 15 percent of one's energy can come from protein. Studies have shown that the addition of a small amount of protein, especially for those training beyond 90 minutes, helps to prevent the body from consuming its own protein from muscles for energy, increases the body's ability to use glucose, and helps to prevent excessive muscle damage. A ratio of 3:1 or 4:1 of carbs to proteins has proven to have the most effective results. Too much protein can delay gastric emptying during exercise and can cause gastrointestinal distress. A range of 8 to 15 grams per hour is a sufficient amount to gain benefits without causing problems.

The sport you participate in and your digestive abilities will determine how and in what forms you supply yourself with these calories. Sports fueling products can be very handy for their convenience as well as their predetermined amounts of carbs to proteins. These come in the form of fluid replacement drinks (hydration and nutrients in one), energy bars, and gels. Gels and bars always require water for better digestion. Some of these products may also contain electrolytes and caffeine. (Hydration and electrolytes will be discussed later in this chapter.) Personally, I tend to avoid the products that contain electrolytes. Everyone has a different sweat rate, which can be affected by ambient air temperature and humidity. There are times when you may need additional electrolytes or calories, but not necessarily both. The combination of the two in pre-made products prevents you from being able to modulate your intake of electrolytes and calories. In addition, the quality of the ingredients in these convenient fueling foods is suspect. Stay away from the simple sugars, food colorings, dyes, and artificial flavorings found in some of these products as best you can, because some of these additives can be very hard for the body to digest and can also lead to other health-related problems. You can create your own products using whole foods. Doing so is worth the extra time, effort, and experimentation for the confidence and results it will provide. Keep in mind that some whole foods can also be hard for the body to digest while active and can require additional water to do so. For long endurance races, whole foods do keep the palate, body, and mind interested with different textures and flavors.

Still, the majority of your fueling should come from liquids. Basically, the best choices and plans will be arrived at as an extension of your training.

The type of fuel you choose will also depend on the type of event you are competing in; you will need to modify your established nutritional program over time and across disciplines. Our bodies are never exactly the same on any given day, nor are the circumstances surrounding our training or competition. Even after 20 years of elite racing experience, endurance athlete Terri Schneider told me how she bonked during her second Western States Ultramarathon and dropped out 20 miles from the finish because she had not figured out her nutrition for that type of event.[11] When Mike Richter entered the world of triathlon and Ironman racing, the three-time Olympian discovered a whole new respect for nutrition and its role in supporting an athlete's endeavors. Not only does each body have different requirements; each sport requires different nutritional support. Athletes I have spoken with tell me about their ongoing process of refining their nutritional plan. Keeping a notebook was a major asset to those who competed on different terrains and in different environments, and they all shared continual education. The most important thing to remember is that your athletic diet during exercise is a delicate balance of choosing the proper fuel and maintaining frequent intake intervals with the goal of preventing breakdowns. (See "Fueling for the Competition" for more on the timing of intake and developing one's nutritional plan.)

Post-Training Nutrition

One of the biggest mistakes an athlete can make is to neglect his or her nutritional program. For those who do pay attention, most concentrate on fueling their bodies during training and competition. Subsequently, the most important part of nutrition, recovery, is neglected. For most athletes who feel as if they have reached a performance plateau, it is this part of their training regime that most likely needs attention. Scientists are discovering that more and more athletes are in a state of overtraining and that both physical and nutritional recovery are keys to greater performance.[12] If you are a successful athlete and you have not yet focused attention on your recovery as a part of your overall nutritional program, imagine the continuing benefits you will get when you do!

Post-training fueling is the most important stage of the nutritional triangle, and its timing is the most critical. A majority of athletes have heard about the post-training "Golden Hour" for nutrient replenishment. I like to use the term "Carbon 15." This term refers to the first 15 minutes post-exercise when an athlete's nutritional recovery should begin. It is the most important time in an athlete's day. Although you may have ceased your active training session, your body is still in a catabolic state wherein the muscles continue to break down protein and are glycogen depleted. Your body also has decreased levels of insulin. Until you begin to consume proper nutrients (carbohydrates and proteins), your body will continue the catabolic process. Hence, the goal of those first 15 minutes post-exercise is to return your body to an anabolic (building) state as soon as possible by taking advantage of the time when your body is best suited for glucose uptake, glycogen synthesis, and protein synthesis. Subsequently, the body will be able to reduce muscle damage, soreness, and breakdown; suppress cortisol; and initiate the recovery process through the release of insulin.

Post-training, most athletes are thinking about resting, showering, cleaning their equipment, picking up the kids, or going back to work, but the first thing you should be thinking of is nutrient intake. The first 15 minutes is the time when your body peaks for its potential to rapidly uptake glucose into the muscles. By the time that Golden Hour is coming to an end, the ability of the body to optimally synthesize glycogen is 40 percent lower. It is immediately post-exercise when your body is most responsive to the effects of insulin; after two hours the muscles can become insulin-resistant. If you do not initiate the replacement process immediately post-exercise—within 45 minutes—your body will not be able to utilize nutrients as effectively. Studies suggest that the body can synthesize glycogen twice as fast during the first hour post-training than at other times and that delaying this replenishment will result in a reduced rate of muscle glycogen storage. The result of not following these steps may include poor performance, muscle soreness, the decreased ability to benefit from training, and possible injury. Complete replenishment can take place over two hours, but one really should begin during the first 15 minutes—Carbon 15. Later, when you do have the time to eat a more substantial meal, those nutrients will be much more effective in the repair and recovery process.

The food you eat in those first 15 minutes can be very simple, and the portions can be small. When the Golden Hour passes, consuming small meals every 30 minutes until you have reached your caloric goal is a great method for continued replenishment. This schedule allows the body to synthesize as much glycogen as possible and prevents hunger and overeating. Remember, pre-training fueling begins with post-training replenishment. This cannot be emphasized enough for those in a continuous training cycle.

The post-training meal comes in many different forms. For some athletes, eating solid foods at this time is the last thing they want to do. This is a normal response because, during exercise, the majority of your body's blood is being diverted to your muscles. Hence, your stomach is yet to have the energy necessary to process solid foods. For others, eating solid foods does not have any adverse affects. Everyone is different. There are a host of sports food products and recovery drinks that are easy to consume, require little preparation (just add water), and are made with the right proportions of nutrients needed post-training. These products also contain micronutrients (electrolytes), macronutrients (amino acids), and antioxidants for complete replenishment. These products do not replace a healthy diet and real food, however.

Those wishing for something a bit more substantial post-training should focus on high-glycemic foods such as raw granola, fruit (banana, raisins, mango, papaya, watermelon, dates) with yogurt or milk, hummus and sprouted bread, or beans, rice, pasta, nut butter and jam. As mentioned earlier, the best protein is whey for its ease of absorption and its amino acid content. Liquids or softer foods are easier for the body to digest and allow the nutrients to get to the muscles faster. Avoiding fats at this time is very important to remember, as they will slow down the ability of the body to absorb the nutrients that it really needs. Make sure to drink adequate amounts of water along with any solid foods that you do consume.

Research varies as to how much carbohydrate and protein one should consume post-training. Carbohydrates and proteins are what the body needs not only to replace what has been used for exercise but also to top off the storage tanks for the next session. Ultimately, it will come down to your individual needs, but there are guidelines to work with. Research done at the University of Texas suggests that the optimal intake for endurance athletes is 1.0 to 1.5 grams carbohydrate per kilogram of body weight (1 kilogram equals 2.2 pounds). Carbohydrates tend to maximize glycogen storage, uptake, and synthesis fastest depending on what the athlete can take. The recommended amount of protein is 0.3 to 0.5 gram per kilogram of body weight. To convert this into calories, you need to multiply each by 4 (each gram of protein and carbohydrate yields approximately 4 calories). Understand that this protein and carbohydrate does not have to be consumed immediately post-training; total

replenishment should take place over the first couple of hours.

Female athletes can have a more difficult time consuming the same amount of carbohydrates as males. The solution for this is not to curb your post-training intake but to take this into account in your overall daily consumption.

The idea behind all of this is to stimulate the production of insulin as quickly as possible because it is responsible for the physiological rebuilding necessary for an athlete's body. The sooner you can begin the process—ideally within 15 minutes—the greater the benefits you will receive. Having sufficient snacks around at all times alleviates the constant need to prepare. Remember, it's important to begin the nutrient consumption with something simple rather than having to wait until your metabolic and recovery opportunity begins to close.

Hydration

Dehydration and depletion of muscle glycogen as a result of a poor nutritional plan are the two main factors that contribute to the body's inability to generate the required energy for exercise. Over 90 percent of the people I speak to who do not finish a race were victims of at least one of these conditions. The same can be said for the folks whose race ends in the medical tent. For most athletes, the primary concern while training or competing is fueling the body with calories in the form of carbohydrates. Although this is a major factor in being able to sustain athletic output, dehydration is the number-one problem that will lead to muscle fatigue and performance breakdown. Hydration should be a big part of your nutritional program and must never be neglected, no matter the training or competing conditions.

Keep in mind that water alone is not hydration and salt itself is not an electrolyte. The two working together will go a long way in improving your training and competitive edge. Hence, the right amount of water intake is more important than all other dietary concerns when it comes to an athlete's nutrition.

There is a reason why water covers over 80 percent of the earth and comprises over 60 percent of our body weight. Water is the element that aids all of the body's most important functions: blood flow and volume, cooling, oxygenation, digestion, and of course, hydration. An athlete's energy primarily comes from stored muscle glycogen and blood glucose that have been converted from carbohydrate. The by-product of using this energy to fuel training sessions is heat. The greater the intensity and duration of exercise, the more heat is produced. The body uses a few mechanisms to dissipate this heat and control its temperature, and without the presence of water these systems fail.

Normal body temperature is 98.6 degrees. Exercising can increase this at varying rates depending on ambient air temperature, weather conditions, exercise factors, and hydration level. What is important to know is that the body's ability to contract muscles becomes compromised when its internal temperature climbs toward 102 degrees. A body temperature above 102 degrees sends signals to our bodies to go into conservation mode, shutting down parts of the physical system. Without a cooling mechanism—water—the core temperature of the body will continue to rise into heat exhaustion and heat stroke, which can result in death.

The chemistry behind this has to do with reduction of blood volume due to lack of water in the body. When exercising, blood is responsible for delivering not only fuel in the form of glycogen to working muscles but also water. Water is also transported just below the surface of the skin so that it can be released through sweat glands, thereby cooling the body. Intense sweating during a workout can account for more than two liters of water loss per hour. When the body is dehydrated, there is a subsequent reduction in the body's blood volume; the body is unable to properly cool itself or deliver oxygen and fuel to working muscles.

Losing water while exercising is inevitable, no matter the weather or how much you sweat. It's how much you lose during any given training session or race that will determine your performance deficit. Attempting to match every ounce of water lost with an equivalent intake is virtually impossible, and it is also unnecessary. Furthermore, doing so could lead to bloating and potentially drinking too much. Maintaining a loss within 1 to 1.5 percent is a good range to aim for. As the gap grows beyond that percentage, heart rate increases, blood volume decreases, and the effects of dehydration become worse.

TABLE 5.2: DETERMINING FLUID AND NUTRIENT NEEDS DURING EXERCISE

Total Caloric Expenditure (calories)	Total Fluid Loss via Sweating (ounces)	Target Carbohydrate Caloric Intake* (calories)	Carbohydrates (grams)	Proteins (grams)	Sports Drink** (ounces)	Water (ounces)	Total Target Fluid Intake (ounces)
200	9	50	12.5	3.1	7	1.9	8.9
250	11	63	15.6	3.9	9	2.4	11.4
300	14	75	18.8	4.7	11	2.9	13.9
350	16	88	21.9	5.5	12	3.4	15.4
450	20	113	28.1	7.0	16	4.4	20.4
500	23	125	31.3	7.8	18	4.8	22.8
550	25	138	34.4	8.6	19	5.3	24.3
600	27	150	37.5	9.4	21	5.8	26.8
650	29	163	40.6	10.2	23	6.3	29.3
700	32	175	43.8	10.9	25	6.8	31.8
750	34	188	46.9	11.7	26	7.3	33.3
800	36	200	50.0	12.5	28	7.8	35.8
850	38	213	53.1	13.3	30	8.2	38.2
900	41	225	56.3	14.1	32	8.7	40.7
1,000	45	250	62.5	15.6	35	9.7	44.7
1,200	54	300	75.0	18.8	42	11.6	53.6

*25 percent of caloric expenditure; **6 percent carbohydrate/1.5 percent protein content

Source: J. Ivy and R. Portman, *The Performance Zone: Your Nutrition Action Plan for Greater Endurance & Sports Performance* (Laguna Beach, CA: Basic Health, 2004), 63. Reprinted by permission of Basic Health Publications, Inc., and J. Ivy.

Determining the correct amount of water to consume is a fairly simple procedure. For most individuals, consuming 20 to 30 ounces of fluid is sufficient. In general, the body sweats about 4.5 ounces of water for every 100 calories expended while exercising. Once you understand how many calories you expend depending on your body weight, intensity, and duration, you can determine your fluid requirements (see Table 5.2).

For example, a 140-pound athlete cycling 15 mph for 45 minutes needs 504 calories for that session. Fluid requirements would be 4.5 times 5 (500 calories divided by 100), or 23 ounces. Adequate rehydration can thus be achieved by consuming 4 to 6 ounces of water every 10 to 15 minutes. This should be something that becomes automatic during your training.

Remember that hydration is part of your overall nutritional strategy as an athlete. Your fluid consumption will only work properly if your body is hydrated before you begin your session, so be sure to keep your fluid intake consistent throughout the day and top off your reserves 20 to 30 minutes before you begin your session. The best way to do this is to consume a sports beverage that has a 6 to 8 percent solution of carbohydrate, thereby simultaneously topping off your body's glycogen levels. Post-training, you want to replace 150 percent of the additional fluids lost during training.

Recording this information in a training and nutrition log, over a substantial period of time, will give you the details necessary to discover your precise needs. The more specific you can be in your entries about your fuel consumption, air temperature, humidity, water temperature, wind, and intensity and duration of each session, the closer you will get to your individual requirements and the better you will be able to prepare for your sport.

Note that while hydration is essential, excess water intake will lead to a condition known as hyponatremia, also referred to as water intoxication, the most serious result of improper fueling. When you consume large amounts of water over the course of a training session without a balance of electrolytes, the sodium in your blood plasma (the liquid part of blood) becomes overdiluted. This happens at the same time your body is sweating and losing salt and minerals. Subsequently, the electrolytes in your body diminish to the point that the functioning of your brain, heart, and muscles causes headaches, nausea, and muscular dysfunction.

Sweating not only causes the body to lose water but also results in a loss of electrolytes. The importance of electrolytes for endurance athletes is fairly easy to understand. First, electrolytes are naturally occurring minerals that when placed in water become conductors for electrical impulses. These electrical impulses are then transferred across cell membranes, providing the necessary stimulus for major bodily functions. The circulatory, respiratory (cardiovascular), nervous, and thermoregulatory systems all rely on electrolytes for their proper functioning. Without them, your heart would not pump, lungs would not expand, muscles would not fire, blood volume would not adapt, sweat glands would not produce, and eventually your brain would cease to function. As such, electrolyte replacement is part and parcel of hydration.

Most athletes believe that electrolyte replacement equates to salt replacement. The majority of electrolytes lost through sweat are sodium (Na) and chloride (Cl), which, of course, are the two elements in table salt. Unfortunately, athletes who rely on products that replace only salt or sodium are missing a number of the other minerals that help support athletic efforts, such as potassium (K), magnesium (Mg), calcium (Ca), phosphate (PO), sulfate (SO), and bicarbonate (HCO). These minerals are responsible for the electrical impulses necessary for your body to function normally; they also add to bone stability and muscle composition. Potassium and sodium are major facilitators of muscle contraction and expansion. Magnesium is highly present throughout the body; 60 to 65 percent of it is found in your bones. In addition, magnesium improves cellular metabolism, smoothes cardiac functioning, and helps stabilize ATP to be broken down into adenosine diphosphate (ADP), reconverted to ATP, and then used as the sole energy source for muscle contraction. Calcium's major role is in bone formation and stability. Without adequate amounts of calcium, stress fractures and osteoporosis are common problems. Calcium also plays a supporting role in muscle contraction, blood coagulation, and electrical impulses. Phosphates are used by muscles to create ATP and creatine phosphate (CP) and when broken down are used as energy. Sulfate and bicarbonate play minor roles for the endurance athlete but are still needed in the body for a balanced electrolyte profile.

When blood volume decreases, the concentration of sodium and chloride in the blood increases. This is what triggers our thirst mechanism. It's important to understand that by the time you are thirsty, your electrolyte balance is already off. These electrolytes need to be replaced to maintain proper muscle function and help prevent cramping. There is debate over the volume of electrolytes that need to be replaced and how much replacement can take place during a training session or race. What is not in debate, however, is that everyone sweats at a different rate and, subsequently, their requirements vary.

Most sports fueling products contain some spectrum of electrolytes, but sweat rates can be affected by the environment as well as the other factors mentioned earlier. Remember, there is no one formula that fits all. For this reason choosing an additional electrolyte product is the best option so as not to increase calories at the same time, as detailed earlier. Obviously the absorption of these is extremely important, so be sure to find ones that are chelated to assist in the uptake process. Experiment, and keep a log of the electrolyte replacement that you use in different weather conditions and at different intensities. If you are working out for long durations—over 90 minutes at a time—and at moderate to high intensities, it is difficult to overconsume electrolytes if you use the suggested guidelines that come with the product. If you have overloaded on electrolytes, you may have swollen hands, wrists, and feet as a result of excessive water retention. This may also lead to some temporary joint discomfort. Underconsumption is a more common condition, resulting in the complications listed above. One clear indicator for me of underconsumption is "growth pains" in my knees. Many people experience this and think it is from overuse, so try experimenting with your electrolyte intake and see if that helps.

One common saying that generally is true is "Prevention is the best medicine." This most certainly applies to hydration. If you wait until your body is already in a state of dehydration, the damage is done and there is no recovering until you stop, rehydrate, and then get back in the game. Here are a few suggestions to help prevent your body from dehydrating:

1. Train your body to adapt to warmer temperatures. This is especially true if you train in a cool climate and compete in a warmer climate. You can reduce your fluid and electrolyte losses by up to 50 percent when you properly train.

2. Instead of drinking plain water, use a sports drink that contains a carbohydrate solution of 6 to 8 percent. You will be able to replace fluids and fuel your body at the same time.

3. Supplement with sodium and electrolytes to help retain fluids and replace the losses incurred from sweating.

4. The day before a long workout or big event, drink two glasses of liquid in addition to what you normally consume.

5. Add juicy fruits to your diet to help boost your water intake.

6. Consume 4 to 10 ounces, depending on your weight, of a sports drink 20 minutes before exercising.

7. Consistently drink 2 to 8 ounces of a sports drink every 10 to 15 minutes while exercising.

8. Drink fluids that are cooler than your body temperature, as they will be more easily absorbed. Replenish between 100 and 150 percent of fluid loss post-training.

Fueling for the Competition

Preparation, confidence, and *performance* are three words that are inextricably linked when it comes to an athlete's big competition day. By then, an athlete has accrued countless hours of training; read dozens of articles on techniques, gear reviews, and nutritional tactics; envisioned his or her race plan; and set some kind of personal goal. At this point, other race-day conditions, such as the weather, are out of your control. There is no more time to experiment or train, so it makes sense to focus on the one element that *can* be controlled: your nutritional fueling. This one piece of the puzzle gives us a belief in our ability and what we can accomplish by having a definitive plan at the start to accomplish our goal. From this confidence you can also make any real-time adjustments to that plan should it be necessary.

Not every competition is a race. It could be rock or ice climbing, a mountain excursion, kayaking, or another sport where the line between training and performing is very thin. The timing of your fuel intake for these events may vary from that of those who are running a race, but the overall guidelines for the quantities remain the same.

Competition-day fueling actually begins the night before. For me, this initiates the final focusing process for the following day. Doing so allows me to get a better night's rest, which can be hard to come by. The night before a race is not the time to experiment with new foods, nor is it the time to load up on carbs.

Your body's ability to uptake glycogen begins weeks before with training and attention to post-training fueling. You certainly want to top off your stores, but overloading the body in an abnormal way can lead to digestive distress.

Sleep is an important part of your race-day fueling. Try to get as much sleep as possible the evening before a race or event and put off eating a full meal unless you can do so 3 hours before you go to bed. Of course, this is easy to say, but how many of us actually sleep through the night before the big day? Most athletes sleep fairly restlessly before a competition. To counter this, make sure you get enough sleep the week leading up to your event and do not rely on that pre-event evening to do so. The goal for the night before is to get an *adequate* amount of sleep. You should have enough event-day adrenaline to overcome a night of tossing and turning and little sleep.

Shifting one's dinner schedule throughout the week before a race will help you and your body adjust to any potential sleep loss and to rising in the very early morning on race day. Dave Scott, six-time Hawaiian Ironman champion, waits 10 hours between dinner and breakfast meals. To get used to this prior to the eve of your event, he suggests adjusting your dinnertime a couple of days before a race. Doing so prevents a shock to your body. Let's say your race will start at 6:30 a.m. You should eat dinner around 5:30 p.m. the day before. This will allow you to eat again around 3:30 a.m., giving you the necessary time to digest the meal before the competition begins.

While you are sleeping, your body burns sugar from blood as well as glycogen from the liver. Given that most people sleep fairly restlessly the night before a race, the body burns even more sugar and glycogen than usual. The race-day morning meal should be medium-sized, 300 to 500 calories, 65 percent carbohydrates, 15 percent proteins, and 20 percent fats. Make sure the meal consists of foods that you know your body will be able to digest easily and will not create problems for you later. Eating at 3:30 in the morning can be difficult or impossible for some and a non-issue for others. A liquid meal, such as a smoothie, is a good idea. You can even go back to bed afterward.

Following the pre-training fueling practices that you have developed is the best approach, whether you eat 3 hours prior to the race or not. About 10 minutes before the start of your race, have a sports fluid replacement drink (approximately 10 ounces, or 100 to 200 calories) or a gel that has a ratio of 3:1 or 4:1 carbohydrate to protein. This will get you through the initial stages of your race. Your next amount of fuel will vary according to the intensity and nature of the sport. Obviously the most limited fueling opportunities will be for swimmers. Ironman and full-distance triathletes can make it through the hour or more it takes to complete the 2.4-mile swim without any intake. Runners, cyclists, climbers, mountaineers, adventure racers, and paddleboarders who have more opportunities to fuel should consider the pre-race boost as the beginning of their fueling plan. For triathletes, especially long-course ones, swimming among hundreds of other competitors for distance can easily offset your body's equilibrium. To allow the body to reset itself, Dave Scott advises his athletes to skip the first aid station between the swim and the bike.

After your event begins, allow your body to calm down from the anticipation and nervous excitement before your next fueling. This should be about 10 to 15 minutes into the race, game, or event. Making conscious stops to take in fuel will go a long way in preventing energy deficits. If you planned your pre-race nutritional intake properly, you will see that you do not need to immediately replace the fuel burned while competing until after the first mile or so.

During the race, you should not attempt to replace every calorie burned with a calorie of fuel. Your body will not be able to assimilate calorie for calorie. The point of fueling is to constantly maintain your engine. Consider yourself a locomotive that already has a fire burning. All you need to do to keep it running is to stoke the fire regularly. Your goal should be to replace 25 to 33 percent of your total calories burned. Trying to do this all at once will only overload your system and smother the fire. Set a schedule for yourself and keep to that schedule throughout the race. You may want to set an alarm on your watch that measures the number of miles you go between fuelings. Plan on refueling every 8 to 15 minutes to start with and then refine this guideline as you gain experience. Your plan also needs to incorporate the varying elements of the event

you are participating in, including terrain and weather conditions, and the sport itself. For example, it is easier for a cyclist to consume fuel than it is for runners. Cyclists have the ability to carry more, and their bodies are not under as much stress as a runner's, although their body position on the bike can create digestive difficulties.

Here are a few things to remember:

1. Build a competition-day nutrition plan and stick to it. Never change your plan within the final few days before a race or event.
2. Know yourself and what works for you.
3. If you run into fueling problems while racing, be flexible with your plan, but don't abandon it. You may need to adjust your timing and quantities, but be careful to avoid grabbing something you may not need at an aid station.
4. Don't ever panic when equipment problems occur. Be willing to readjust your goals and leave your ego at home. The primary goal is to finish the race safely.
5. Be confident in the choices you have made.
6. Have fun!

The Right Gear to Carry Your Fuel

When there is gear involved, even nutrition can have its fun side. As race day approaches, the hours of hard training and mental fatigue slowly ease and are replaced by excitement and anticipation. All of your work will finally be put to the test. Your nutritional plan should be well thought out and established. This means having a solid understanding of what fuel you are going to use, how much, and when. Choosing the gear to carry your fuel—and, for some, to prepare along the way—is just as important. Most athletes pride themselves on being on the cutting edge when it comes to knowing and owning the fastest, lightest gear the sports industry has to offer. Unfortunately, this knowledge generally does not extend into the area of nutrition or, until recently, in consideration of the environment. Knowing what to eat and drink is one thing, but being able to efficiently and conveniently transport it while training or competing is another. Because your fueling plan is individualized, do not rely on the race organizers to have your particular fueling products on hand at aid and water stations.

Racecourses have well-positioned aid stations, but carrying your own fuel is standard for most athletes. As a result, most athletes will be taking only water from the kind volunteers who staff the aid stations (always thank these folks as you pass by). For long-course races, having a combination of liquid (fluid replacement drinks), gels, and bars is recommended for self-support. Those who have the ability to carry more or have crew support, such as mountaineers, backcountry skiers and snowboarders, paddleboarders, adventure racers, and ultramarathoners, may choose to carry a variety of whole foods.

Events and races can be a veritable disaster for the environment. The abundance of plastic water bottles, wrappers, and nonrecyclable items can give any sport a black eye. Do what you can to limit the usage of unnecessary items such as food wrappers, and choose gear and products from companies that use recycled and environmentally sensitive materials in their products and that are conscious about their impact on the earth. Unfortunately, few companies currently use such practices, but your purchasing power can impress others to follow suit. GoLite is a prime example of how a company can be responsible by purchasing renewable energy credits and CO_2 offsets through NativeEnergy (www.nativeenergy.com). GoLite was able to offset 100 percent of its greenhouse emissions for 2007 and 2008 as a result of company operations. Mountainsmith is also leading the way in environmentally conscientious outdoor gear production. A number of its items are made from 100 percent recycled materials and others are free of polyvinyl chloride (PVC). (The use of PVC in plastics and other materials is known to be toxic to the environment.) Amphipod is contributing to this effort in small part by making the bottles for its fuel belts free of bisphenol-A (BPA). The gel flasks, water bottles, and hydration bladders from Ultimate Direction, FuelBelt, and Nathan Sports are all BPA-free as well. (Studies have shown levels of BPA in humans with health problems, such as immune system malfunction, cancer, mammary gland issues, and prostate issues.) The impact that one individual and the disposal of his or her gear can have on the environment in just one day can last beyond his or her lifetime.

Although there are not as many options for carrying fuel as there are fueling products, more are becoming available as the importance of nutrition to overall athletic health has been recognized. Personal preference is, again, a factor in the nutritional gear that you use. Different sports have different requirements, and there are many variables to consider when making a purchase. As with the fueling aspect of your plan, there is going to be some trial and error with your nutritional gear. A water bottle, hydration pack, or fuel belt might work for someone else, but when you actually put it to the test, the keys to its success are comfort, ease of use, aerodynamic properties, efficiency, durability, capacity, stability, and, most important, access.

The day has yet to come when I have seen someone swim with a hydration pack, and because the only "floating aid stations" I've been to serve margaritas, it's the land-based sports that require carrying fuel. I have divided them into categories, but keep in mind the overlaps and sharing of gear and information between sports.

Gear for Triathletes, Road Cyclists, and Mountain Bikers

If your fuel and hydration source is difficult to access, you won't use it, and, in time, you will forget that it is there. For cyclists racing on a time-trial or tri-bike, and mountain bikers who have water bottles attached to the frame of their bikes, it can be hazardous to continu-

ally look down and reach for those bottles. The aero water bottle was invented for cyclists who need a front-mounted hydration system. These low-profile bottles can be attached between your aerobars or to your bike's frame. They are easy to refill—because they do not have caps—and having them right in front of your face means you never have to take your hands off your handlebars to drink; moreover, it is impossible to forget to hydrate because the straw is inches from your lips. The difference in the designs of aero bottles is in how they attach to aerobars. When choosing a design, make sure it can be adapted for clip-on or stationary bars and can be adjusted for width. The two most common are made by Syntace (www.syntace.com), which offers the Jetstream NXT, and Profile Design (www.profile-design.com). PodiumQuest (www.podiumquest.com) also makes a front-mounted hydration system that has two separate chambers, which can hold different liquids.

Depending on your bike's frame and your personal choice, mounting water bottles behind the saddle is another option for triathletes. Personally, I find saddle-mounted bottles a bit cumbersome, but you may want to give them a try. Depending on how many you carry—one or two—and how full they are, the setup can affect a bicycle's weight distribution and its performance during a race. Some models, like those from XLAB and Profile Design, integrate spare tubes and CO_2 cartridges. In a class of its own is NeverReach (www.neverreach.com), which offers a system that eliminates the need to reach behind for a drink by running a tube from its rear-mounted bottles to your handlebars. These bottles and tubes carry a whopping 64 ounces of fluid. PK Racing did some testing of this product when it was full of liquid and actually found it to improve riding times. Your riding terrain will determine how much fluid you want to hold and how best to access it.

Riding with a hydration pack is the best option for those who ride off-road. A cyclist is able to carry additional food and gear in these packs. Detailed attention should be paid to the design of these packs so that they fit well, distribute body heat and weight evenly, and are accessible. Nathan Sports (www.nathansports.com) offers a number of designs to choose from, including one designed specifically for women. The GoLite (www.golite.com) Fusion is another multiuse pack suitable for off-road bike riding.

Cyclists out for longer distances tend to invent their own devices rather than use what's on the market. When carrying fuel other than water, a jersey with pockets generally does the trick. Triathlon jerseys tend to have fewer and shallower pockets. I have seen bike frames adorned with energy gels taped all over and tri-shorts bulging with whatever they can hold. This can be uncomfortable and have an impact on aerodynamics, and these packets can become hard to handle when they are wet with sweat.

The Bento Box (www.tniusa.com) is the original bike lunch box. Made from lightweight nylon mesh, it attaches to the frame or stem of your bike, affording easy access and plenty of space to carry gels, bars, or other snacks.

TNiUSA also makes pockets that can be attached between your aerobars that hold a water bottle and fuel or just fuel alone. Nathan Sports has a version of the Bento Box called the Feed Bag, and Epic Ride Research has made one specifically for mountain biking. The boxes also provide a space to carry used wrappers instead of tossing them on the racecourse, which should *not* be an option. Two tips: if using bars or sandwiches, cut them up into smaller pieces so you can handle them easily, and pre-open gel packs.

If gels are your preferred fueling choice, a mounted gel flask carrier is an excellent way to go. Positioned on your top tube or stem, it is easy to reach and hard to forget. If one flask of fuel is not enough for your ride or you like to carry different flavors, put an additional flask in your pocket. These flasks eliminate having to open gel packs on the road and are garbage-free and course-friendly. Buying gels in bulk containers goes one step further, as does making your own, in not adding to the waste stream of garbage with all of the packaging. Nathan Sports, Ultimate Direction (www.ultimate direction.com), FuelBelt, and GuSports sell gel flasks.

Another option for carrying gels, concentrated powder mix, or a home mixture is a regular water bottle. One water bottle can hold a lot of gels. The trick here is to add a gel along with some water and then mark portions on the bottle with a permanent marker. This way you can monitor your consumption throughout your ride. Just remember to shake the bottle well before taking a sip. The same holds true for other types of fuel, or if you want to make a concentrate. Try to mark the bottle on a per serving basis that allows you to be mindful of your consumption. I have found this approach to be very handy for monitoring my intake while also refocusing my mind when it wanders by giving it a task to keep it sharp. It's a great way to carry what you need. Just don't drop it!

There are not many options for carrying electrolyte pills. Some people dispense what they think they will need into their fuel, but that does not allow much flexibility for variable conditions. Another option is those little rubber purses that Grandma used to hold her coins. You can stash them in your Bento Box or pocket and be satisfied, but these are not very waterproof and can be difficult to handle. I have seen and tried a few homemade get-ups but none seem to be as clever as the SaltStick (www.saltstick.com). If you like gadgets, these nifty dispensers are certain to please. They come in two sizes: a mini size that fits inside drop-down bars and a larger size that is made for TT, mountain, and tri bikes.

The fuel belt is another good option for triathletes. The company FuelBelt (wwwfuelbelt. com) coined the term and created a product category that other companies have since entered. The basic design of fuel belts allows one to carry fuel and hydration in flasks that attach to a waist belt. How these flasks are attached as well as the number of flasks differentiate one belt from another. Thankfully, the ultra-running community has brought out improved versions that rival the standard belt. Because carrying fuel at your waist can be cumbersome, it's important to test several fuel belts before buying. No fuel belt is completely perfect—or bounce-free—but companies have improved the designs considerably.

I used the original FuelBelt in a number of races and had plenty of success. The company has since updated the FuelBelt's design with cord locks and flask straps that are supposed to minimize shifting. The belt that seems to be the most versatile is the Amphipod (www. amphipod.com), which gives the wearer the ability to choose how many flasks to carry (up to five) and where and how to place them—vertically, horizontally, or upside down. The flasks hold fuel or hydration, and there are add-on accessories such as a pouch, pockets, and race number tabs. The flasks can be removed and replaced with a bit of practice and are comfortable to carry. These belts work well on individuals with large body frames or those who like extra padding and protection. The downside is that the belts can be bulky. Nathan Sports (www.nathansports.com) makes Elite/Race and Race/Speed belts that do not have the versatility of the Amphipod belts but position the flask carriers in a way conducive to running and are easily accessible. The individual flasks hold 10 ounces of fluid and are easy to remove and replace. I find that the fuel belts that carry three or more flasks make it hard to maintain even weight distribution after one flask is empty, so I always try to alternate drinking from each flask to keep the weight comfortable. It is crucial to train with a fuel belt if you are going to use one when you compete.

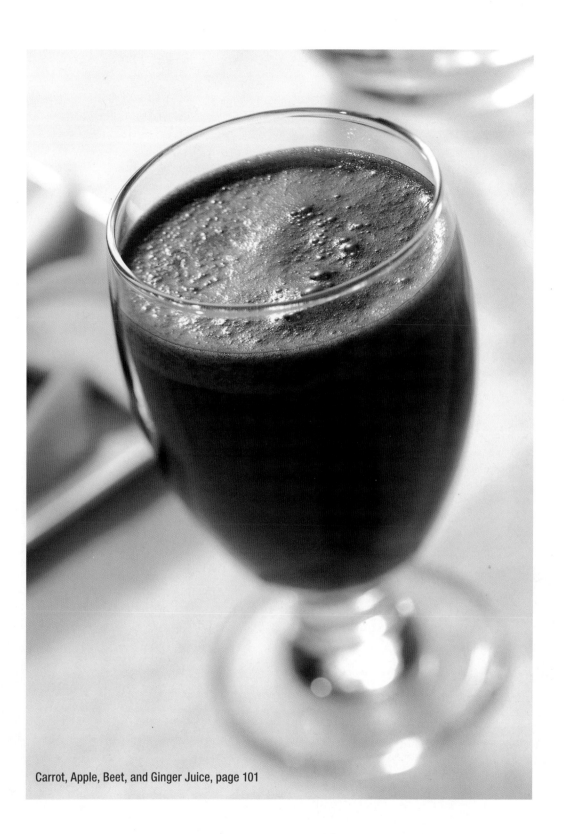

Carrot, Apple, Beet, and Ginger Juice, page 101

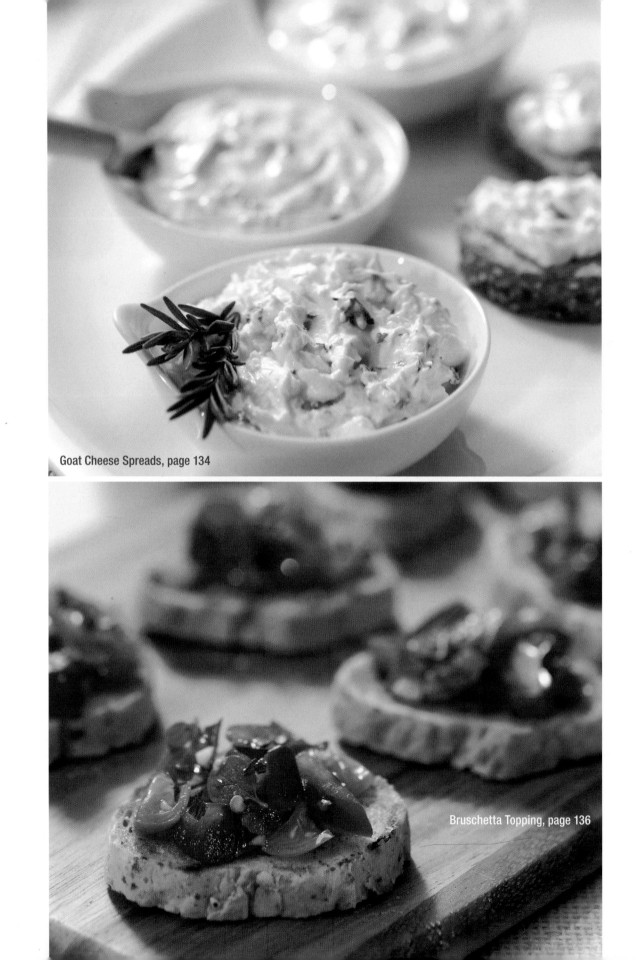

Goat Cheese Spreads, page 134

Bruschetta Topping, page 136

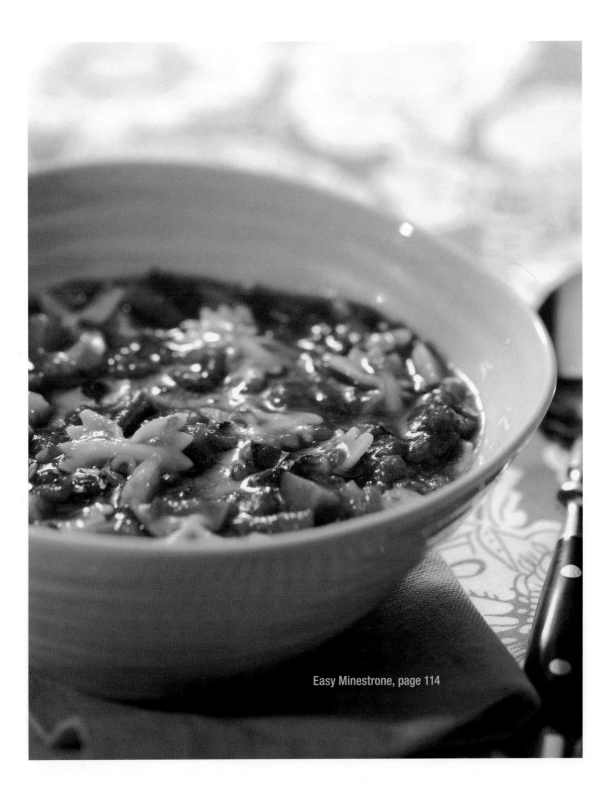

Easy Minestrone, page 114

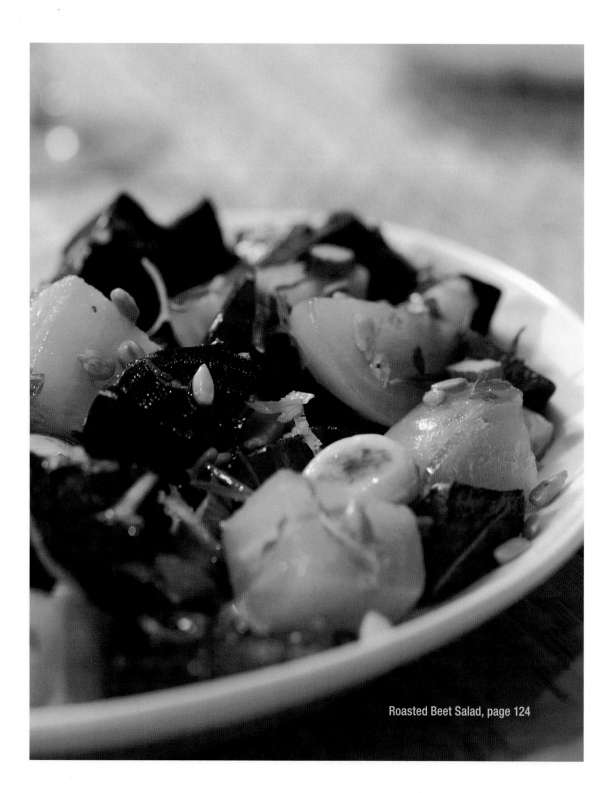

Roasted Beet Salad, page 124

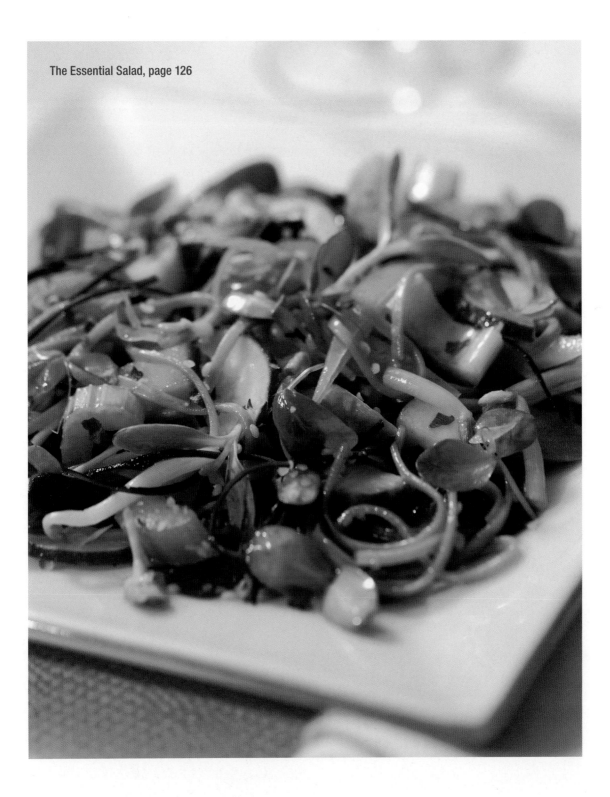

The Essential Salad, page 126

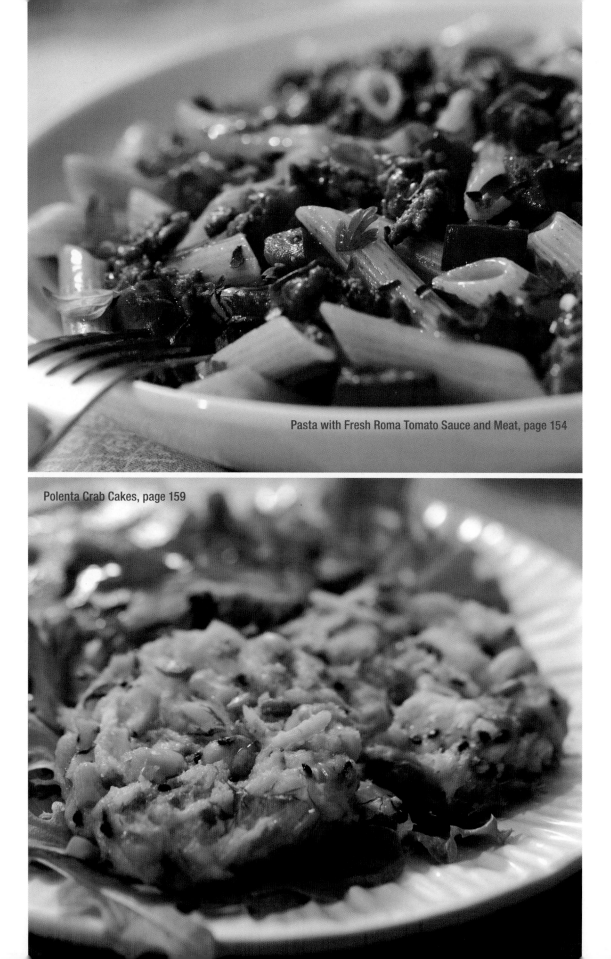

Pasta with Fresh Roma Tomato Sauce and Meat, page 154

Polenta Crab Cakes, page 159

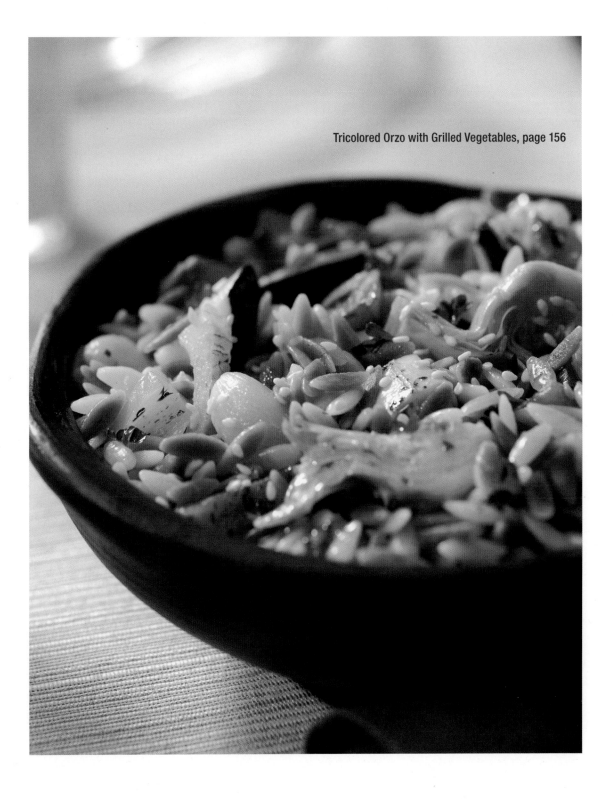
Tricolored Orzo with Grilled Vegetables, page 156

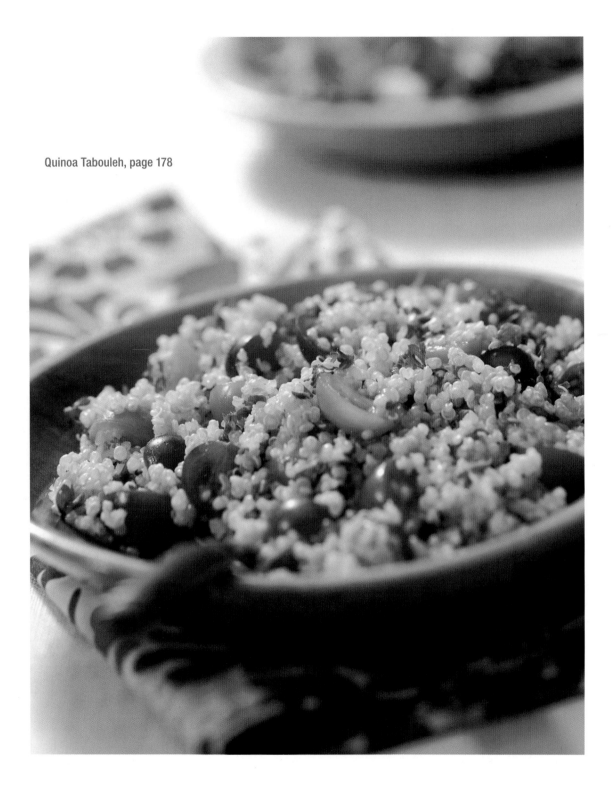

Quinoa Tabouleh, page 178

Gear for Adventure Racers,
Ultramarathoners, Cross-Country/
Backcountry Skiers, Snowboarders,
and Trail Runners

The primary considerations when running, skiing, or racing long distances are storage capacity, comfort, and access while on the move. For the most part, the options are a backpack or a waist pack. As mentioned above, the weight and bounce factor of waist packs can be very uncomfortable. The GoLite HydroSprint is a streamlined design that does not allow you to carry additional items but is excellent for middle-distance trail running or in a race where you can get refills from aid stations or a crew. Ultimate Direction has a line of trail waist packs, such as the Katoa, for low-impact and flatter terrain. The Buzz II from Mountainsmith also fits into this middle-distance category and is made from recycled materials.

A backpack is for adventure racers and ultramarathoners who need to carry hydration, food, and a change of clothes. Trail runners can take advantage of backpacks that have been streamlined for shorter distances. Ultimate Direction has a series of backpacks starting with a small version, known as the Wasp, up through the larger Hornet. Nathan Sports has divided its packs into Race Vests and Bladder Paks. GoLite's Adrenaline series includes a small day model and another suitable for multiday adventure racing.

There are times when adventure racers, trail runners, and cross-country skiers travel far enough that they need to stop to cook, rather than get their nutritional fueling on the run. They need gear that is light, durable, and easy to use. Primus has a great compact, all-in-one stove in its ETApacklite. It's an easy canister-fueled setup that incorporates cooking pots directly into its construction. The canisters are recyclable, and the stove is heat-efficient, cooking quickly and with little fuel waste.

In the life of an endurance athlete, food and water availability post-workout or post-race is all part of the nutritional protocol. These days there is gear for transporting and preparing all manner of fuel. It's as important to understand the quality and impact on the environment of these items as it is the food you put in them. Stainless steel is the safest on-the-go option. Primus makes a set of stainless-steel cookware for the green gourmet that is a departure from the unhealthy aluminum ones that were the former lightweight standard. The stainless-steel set, which is best for those camping on backcountry excursions, is easy to clean, heats fast and evenly, and retains heat to reduce fuel use. The cookware is not super-thick, though, so be careful on high-powered stoves. Primus also has some great stainless-steel food storage containers and water bottles that keep food items hot or cold for hours and will not leach chemicals. The Primus Atle BBQ stove is a great item for those camping out before an event. Unlike standard camp stoves, this one combines a burner and a grill into one unit and does not sacrifice size. The grill side can also be used as another burner. Mountainsmith even has a PVC-free cooler that is great for bringing food along to races, training, or for crews needing to carry stuff from the road.

Nathan Sports makes reusable stainless-steel water bottles in various sizes that are better not only for your health but also for the environment. Each year millions of water bottles end up in landfills because they have not been recycled properly. Refilling a water bottle will reduce that impact dramatically as well as keep you from ingesting harmful chemicals that could leach into your food or water supply.

It is crucial to understand that your gear is as important as the nutrition it will carry. Be sure to train with your gear regularly so you are familiar and comfortable with how it works on race day. Good luck, and see you at the race!

6

Recipes

For me, cooking is a passion. I love every part of it, from shopping and prepping to cleaning up—and imagining the possibilities of what can be done with the leftovers. Cooking—and enjoying the good food that you cook—is the daily reward for your efforts in your training and racing. Cooking also forms the bridge between your nutrition and lifestyle, the place where your food and eating choices express themselves in the decisions about your quality of life. My hope is that you will find joy and inspiration as you read and use these recipes, and that they will become a stepping-stone toward your own creativity and fulfillment in your kitchen.

Preparing delicious, nutritious food does not require you to be an accomplished chef. You need only a willingness to learn and experiment and a desire to provide yourself with the best possible base for your athletic performance.

Every athlete at the top of his or her game understands the importance of nutrition. Jamie Mitchell, Australia's seven-time champion of the world's most grueling paddleboard race—32 miles across the channel from Molokai to Oahu, Hawaii—told me, "Physical training has its limits. The refinement of that work comes with nutrition."[1] Needless to say, Jamie does almost all of his own cooking. And he is not the only one; from world-class snowboarder Nicolas Muller to Ironman champion Dave Scott, great athletes participate in the preparation of their own meals. Let these recipes become the foundation of your nutrition, a fundamental piece of your training program, and the fuel for doing the things you love to do.

Getting Started

The recipes in this chapter are a departure from the gourmet, celebrity, and restaurant chef's intricate repertoire, which is rarely compatible with an athlete's everyday routine and active lifestyle. These recipes are designed to be simple to execute, yet they are wholesome, flavorful, and, most important, contain the full spectrum of nutrients necessary to support the daily energy requirements of an active lifestyle. They are contemporary recipes based on traditional techniques modified to support the pace of modern living. Most of them are also quick to prepare, and many can be thrown together on the spur of the moment or easily whipped together after rigorous hours of training.

All of these recipes are made with ingredients that are easy to find in farmers' markets, local natural food stores, or local grocery stores. If necessary, the ingredients can also be sourced via the Internet (see the "Resources" chapter in this book). You will also find that prepared or cooked ingredients for one recipe can be refrigerated or frozen for use in other recipes. Buying a bunch of herbs, a head of broccoli, or a container of spices and using only a portion for a single recipe is a waste of money, and it can leave you uninspired, discouraged, and frustrated wondering what to do with the rest. Although it is important to prepare food with fresh ingredients, the recipes also incorporate leftovers, which saves precious time and avoids waste.

Many of the recipes have interchangeable parts. For example, a dressing or marinade for one can easily be used in another. The recipes can also be doubled or halved without affecting their integrity. The goal is to nurture your culinary and personal intuition so that cooking becomes a seamless part of your active life that supports your body's nutritive requirements.

The recipes also depart from the everyday methods of conventional cooking and eating in that they blend organic, raw, fermented, soaked, and cooked foods in an approach that I have perfected and used as a complement to my own training and lifestyle, as well as for other athletes. However, they are not puffed up with ingredients that are hard to find or techniques that are difficult to master. They were created for people living active lives.

Let me caution you: these recipes are not designed to turn you into a chef. Rather, they have been designed by a chef—who is also an athlete devoted to a nutritionally balanced diet and sustaining the environment of this earth—to help you eat more nutritionally. I have gathered these flavorful recipes from around the world. They are full of tastes and secrets I learned in small kitchens in Thailand, talking to street vendors in Indonesia, and watching women in India carefully choose their spices. They also blend my formal culinary education and restaurant training with personal farmwork and my study of traditional societies combined with an environmentally preservationist approach to fulfilling the nutritional requirements of a busy athletic lifestyle.

Methods and Guidelines

There are a few guidelines for food preparation that will help you master the recipes in this book.

Always read the recipe from start to finish before beginning to prepare. This might seem obvious, but it's worth keeping in mind every time you approach a new recipe, whether in this book or elsewhere. Reading the recipe through allows you to imagine the cooking process. You will be able to visualize what you are going to need, which will save time once you get started.

Get your ingredients together before you start cooking. Look over the ingredients and portion them per the recipe.

Focus all of your attention on the execution of the recipe. Cooking is a series of successive steps, and the point at which it all comes together is where you have to be the most "present." This is the point at which you transfer your love and appreciation for the ingredients into the meal that you are preparing. Without getting too esoteric or mystical, let me say that cooking is a very energetic process. Try cooking the same meal when you are filled with joy and again when you are filled with anger. Your energy changes the way the food will taste.

Taste everything along the way. This is one of the most important parts of cooking. Begin tasting when you purchase your ingredients and continue until you are about to take the pan off the stove or pour a drink from a blender. Continual tasting will enhance your culinary intuition, making you aware of flavor subtleties, the quality and freshness of ingredients, and how flavors change when foods are cooked and paired with other ingredients. Cooking is not just a relationship between you and the food but also among the ingredients themselves.

Never make a meal only of cooked foods. Each of the recipes relies on the principle that any cooked food should be paired with something raw, such as sprouted seeds or nuts, very lightly blanched or steamed veggies, fresh greens or sprouts, or fruits or vegetables that have been lacto-fermented. Incorporating raw foods will reduce the amount of time you spend cooking as well as provide your body with live enzymes and nutrients that will aid in digestion and absorption.

Use your resources. If you always think in terms of conserving energy, you will always be one step ahead. If you have a pot of water boiling for pasta or noodles, for example, repurpose the water in that pot to blanch or steam veggies or fish. When the oven is in use for one thing, put something else in there to take advantage of the residual heat. This approach might add a bit more time to what you are presently doing (though it usually doesn't), but it will definitely save time later.

Use the steam-sauté method instead of a lot of oil. Who says oil and water don't mix? They do when you are looking for flavor and healthy cooking. Cooking oils, especially those that are polyunsaturated, can become rancid when they are heated. To avoid using more oil than is needed, I "steam-sauté." In a pan, I flavor the oil with some garlic, ginger, or onion, typically toss in some quickly blanched veggies, and then add some of the hot water that was used to blanch the vegetables. This creates steam and, as the water evaporates, a sauce.

Use organic ingredients and raw products, and buy locally. All of the recipes are based upon the tenets in this book. Although the recipes may not specifically say so, you can correctly assume that they all depend on organic ingredients sourced as locally as possible, and that products such as oils, vinegars, butters, honey, cheese, and so forth are raw.

Soaking and Sprouting Nuts, Seeds, and Grains

Lost in the advent of modern equipment for cooking and refrigeration were the techniques and appreciation for soaking and sprouting grains, nuts, and seeds. Lost, but not forgotten. Thanks to those who have studied traditional and healthy methods of food preparation, we can re-create these techniques and enhance the nutrient quality of our foods while revitalizing and restoring our bodies.

As we know, nature has a very well-organized and self-regulating system of sustainability of space and resources. Nuts, seeds, and grains have essential nutrients that turn them into plants. But, like all living things, they need the proper environment to grow and nurture.

As a protective mechanism to delay premature germination and release of their nutrients, nuts, seeds, legumes, and grains contain antinutrients or enzymes as well as phytic acid. In fact, the phytic acid in these plants will bind to magnesium, iron, calcium, copper, and zinc in the body and actually prevent their absorption, thus creating deficiencies of minerals that are vital to the body, especially for the athlete. Enzyme specialist Dr. Edward Howell noted that consuming raw nuts and seeds neutralizes our bodies' own enzymes in the digestive tract, subsequently preventing nutrient assimilation and digestibility, as well as causing a swelling of the pancreas.[2] But there is a very simple solution to this. Soaking and/or sprouting seeds, grains, and flour in acidified warm water (just plain water for sprouting) or milk, and soaking nuts in salted water, will deactivate the enzyme inhibitors, as well as phytic acid, by mimicking the environment that promotes their growth. In doing so, the nutrients become much more bio-available. The only seed that does not contain enzyme inhibitors is hemp. The hemp seed does contain edestin, however, which according to David Wolfe is "perhaps the most bio-available form of protein."[3]

Once grains, flours, or legumes have been soaked, they can then be used for cooking. Seeds as well as most legumes can be sprouted into tiny shoots and then eaten raw in salads and added to sandwiches, wraps, and spring rolls. Once nuts have been soaked, it is best to then dry them to prevent spoilage.

Soaking and sprouting are easy processes. There are many types of "sprouters" on the

TABLE 6.1. SPROUTING AND SOAKING TIMES

Variety	Dry Measure*	Soaking Time**	Sprouting Time	Length at Harvest
Alfalfa seeds	¼ cup	8 hours	5 days	1 inch
Azuki beans	1 cup	12 hours	3–4 days	1 inch
Broccoli seeds	1 cup	8 hours	5–7 days	1 inch
Chickpeas	1 cup	12 hours	3–4 days	¾ inch
Clover seeds	1 cup	8 hours	5 days	1 inch
Lentils	1 cup	12 hours	3–4 days	½ inch
Mung beans	½ cup	12 hours	3–4 days	1–2 inches
Radish seeds	¼ cup	8 hours	5 days	1 inch
Sunflower seeds	2 cups	6 hours	1–2 days	3 inches

*Per half-gallon jar
**Can be soaked overnight

market (see "Resources"), or you can use a mason jar and a piece of cloth. Refer to Table 6.1 for sprouting and soaking times.

Another way to enhance digestibility and nutrient content is through lacto-fermentation, which has the added benefit of not requiring refrigeration for storage. See the sauerkraut recipe for a more detailed explanation of its benefits and usage.

Easy at-Home Sprouting Instructions
1. Place seeds or beans in half-gallon jar, fill with water, and cover with cheesecloth or other mesh fabric, securing with a rubber band.
2. Soak for prescribed time at room temperature and drain.
3. Rinse seeds/beans with fresh water and drain every 8–12 hours for the suggested amount of days or until the sprouts are of the desired length.
4. Set jar at 45-degree angle, tilting it to rest on a small bowl, to drain the rest of the water.
5. Give final rinse, drain as in step 4, and store in refrigerator.

Soaking and Dehydrating Nuts
Nuts generally cannot be sprouted to the point where they grow a visible appendage. On occasion one might find a nub emerging from a skinless almond or peanut, but that's it. To increase the enzymatic activity of nuts and to neutralize their nutrient inhibitors, however, they can be germinated by soaking in fresh water. During his research into enzyme activity and sprouting, Dr. Edward Howell witnessed squirrels burying nuts and then returning to

them once they had germinated.[4] Although the germination is not always visible, enzymatic activity is improved.

Soaking times for nuts vary from a half hour to three days; Table 6.2 shows recommendations for some common varieties. Note that nuts with a high fat content, such as macadamia and brazil nuts, do not benefit from germination.

After soaking, nuts should be dried (dehydrated) at temperatures around 115 degrees. Having a dehydrator makes this easy; simply follow the manufacturer's directions. To use an oven, set the temperature below "warm." Use an oven thermometer, placed inside, to monitor the temperature. Place nuts on a sheet tray lined with parchment paper and put it on the top rack of the oven. Shake the tray from time to time for even drying and to accelerate the process.

TABLE 6.2: SOAKING TIMES FOR NUTS

Variety	Soaking Time*
Almonds	2–3 days
Cashews	2 hours
Filberts	12 hours
Peanuts	2–3 days
Pecans	6 hours
Pine nuts	30 minutes–1 hour
Walnuts	24 hours

*Can be soaked overnight

JUICES & SMOOTHIES

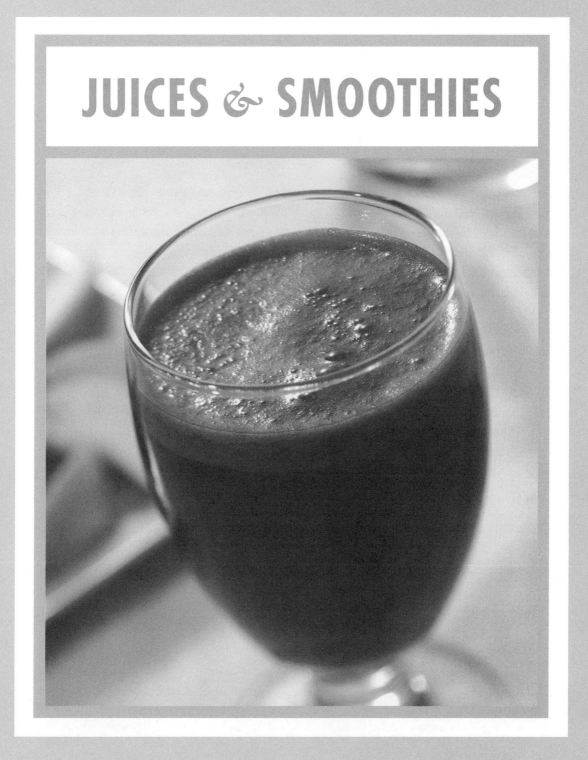

JUICES

Freshly made juices are among the most uplifting, energetic, and nutrient-packed foods available. When I conduct detox and fasting programs, I specify that juices be the only food consumed for a week or more. Juices require very little time to prepare, and most mechanical juicers are easy to use and clean. Preparing your own juices is also a great way to use up vegetables and herbs that may be left over from other recipes. Whether you are starting your day, on the go, or just looking for a light meal, a fresh juice is a fantastic way to fuel your body.

Juicers separate the pulp or solid material of the fruit, vegetable, or herb from the liquid and its nutrients. Hence, the quality of the produce is essential to the quality of the juice. Fresh and organic is the only way to go!

There are endless varieties of juice combinations but my starting point is fresh, local, and in-season ingredients. The recipes here blend that approach with nutritional guidance to put together juices that taste great, make sense, and are healthy.

Different juicers extract differently, so the recipes here are guidelines. Use your imagination and palate to help you determine the right proportions.

Carrot, Apple, Beet, and Ginger Juice

SERVES 1

This is the classic "beginner's" juice because of its sweetness, great flavor, and colors! It is also packed with nutrients and makes for a great pick-me-up. The sweet apple makes it kid-friendly as well.

Beets are strong blood and liver detoxifiers. I have seen people drinking juices that were too heavy on beets become lightheaded because their bodies could not process the toxins as quickly as they were being released. For this reason, and also to help balance the sweetness of this drink, I sometimes add half of a lemon to the recipe.

2–3 large carrots
1 apple (I like to use Granny Smith apples, but Gala,
    Empire, or any local variety is also good)
½ inch fresh gingerroot
½ medium-sized beet

PREPARATION

Put all ingredients through your juicer.
Pour into a tall glass and enjoy.

VARIATION

If the juice is too sweet for you, add the juice of a lemon.

Pineapple, Cucumber, Ginger, and Mint Juice

SERVES 1

Pineapple yields a lot of sweetness, so I add cucumber to balance it out.

2 cups pineapple, with rind
1 medium cucumber
½ inch fresh gingerroot, peeled
½ cup packed fresh mint (with stems)

PREPARATION

Put all ingredients in a juicer. Pour into a tall glass and enjoy.

How to peel and slice ginger

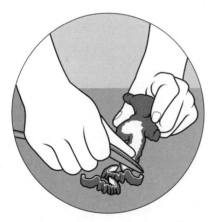

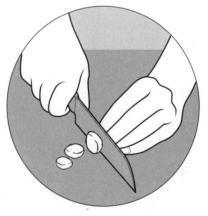

1. Using flat edge of a spoon, scrape skin off ginger in short downward motions until flesh is revealed.

2. Using kitchen knife, slice across fibrous grain with small cuts.

Pear, Kale, Parsley, and Celery Juice

SERVES 1

This is a great post-workout drink; the folate in the greens will aid in cell maintenance and repair as well as amino acid metabolism, which in turn will help with muscle recovery.

1 whole Anjou or Bosc pear
3 leaves green kale (or lacinato kale or green chard)
1 bunch parsley
2 stalks celery

PREPARATION

Rinse all ingredients, pop them into a juicer, and enjoy.

Watermelon, Ginger, Lime, and Mint Juice

SERVES 1

Watermelon is one of the few foods rich in lycopene. Studies show that watermelon has 40 percent more lycopene than an equal amount of raw tomatoes and is loaded with vitamins A, B6, and C. In addition, watermelon is a great source of potassium, which regulates fluids and mineral balance in our bodies, protects against high blood pressure, and prevents muscle cramps. For all of these reasons, I make a big jug of this and leave it in my fridge for any time during the day and especially before and after workouts.

My juicer works better on fruits that have less water content, so for juices with watermelon I always re-strain the pulp extract through cheesecloth.

2 cups watermelon, rind removed
½ inch fresh gingerroot
½ lime
½ cup packed fresh mint with stems

PREPARATION

Put all ingredients through your juicer. Strain through cheesecloth. Pour into a tall glass and enjoy.

VARIATIONS

- Add cilantro (¼ cup of cilantro with stems) in place of or in addition to the mint. Cilantro adds a great flavor and is also a heavy-metal detoxifier.
- Substitute a radish or 2 for the gingerroot to add just a bit of spice and to get its great blood-alkalizing properties.

SMOOTHIES

Athletes have an unfortunate tendency to view smoothies as vehicles for protein and other "energy" powders and supplements. These additions can have their benefits if used to enhance your diet, but they can also turn basic, nutritious smoothies into huge mixes of a lot of calories and too much protein. Smoothies shouldn't be a substitute for whole foods; I've noticed that they often leave me with the feeling of a hollow, empty stomach not long after consumption, at which point I find myself craving something more substantial. As a result, they can become a big part of your daily calories and a cause of overeating.

However, smoothies can also serve a purpose when used as easily digestible foods that can be quickly prepared before and after training. They're especially good for early morning sessions, and the recipes here will provide a good energy boost without overloading your system.

Banana-Tahini Delight

SERVES 1

1 large banana

1 tablespoon raw tahini or almond, cashew, or walnut butter

1 tablespoon raw honey or pure maple syrup

1 tablespoon raw coconut butter

1 cup cold water

3 ice cubes (about 1 cup of crushed ice)

PREPARATION

Blend all ingredients in a blender until smooth. Pour into a tall glass and enjoy.

Coconut Almond Smoothie

SERVES 1

Coconut water is nature's ultimate sports beverage, with a spectrum of electrolytes that mimics the human body's. It is easily digested and absorbed and contains medium-chain triglycerides, a good endurance source. Coconut water is best when fresh, but it can also be purchased in juice boxes, though sources with preservatives should be avoided.

12 ounces coconut water
½ cup fresh coconut meat or 1 heaping tablespoon raw coconut butter
1 small banana
1 tablespoon raw almond butter
1 tablespoon hempseed powder
2 teaspoons raw honey, agave, or pure maple syrup

PREPARATION

Put all ingredients in blender and blend until smooth. Pour into a tall glass and enjoy.

SunPower Greens Smoothie

SERVES 1

This is about as complete as a drink gets for an athlete: raw healthy fats, micronutrients, greens, antioxidants, and protein, as well as minerals, electrolytes, fiber, and adrenal gland support. This is truly power from the sun.

8–12 ounces fresh coconut water

½ cup raw coconut flesh or 1 heaping tablespoon raw coconut butter

½ tablespoon maca root powder*

1 tablespoon SunPower Greens**

½ cup blueberries, raspberries, or strawberries, fresh or frozen

1 tablespoon raw hempseed powder

1 tablespoon raw honey

1 tablespoon raw pumpkin seeds, sprouted

1 small banana (optional)

PREPARATION

Put all ingredients in blender and blend until smooth. Pour into a tall glass and enjoy.

*Maca root grows in the high plateaus of Peru's Andean mountains, 13,000–15,000 feet above sea level, where it has been used for centuries as a staple of the native diet and for medicinal remedies. Maca is known as an adaptogen, similar to licorice, ginseng, and holy basil, helping to increase the body's resistance to stress, trauma, anxiety, and fatigue. Maca contains two of three essential fatty acids (oleic and linoleic) and has a complex amino acids profile containing a total of eighteen amino acids, including seven of the nine essential amino acids. Maca contains 60–75 percent carbohydrate, 10–14 percent protein, 8.5 percent fiber, and 2.2 percent lipids, a perfect combination for athletes and active lifestyles.

**My product, available from my website.

SOUPS

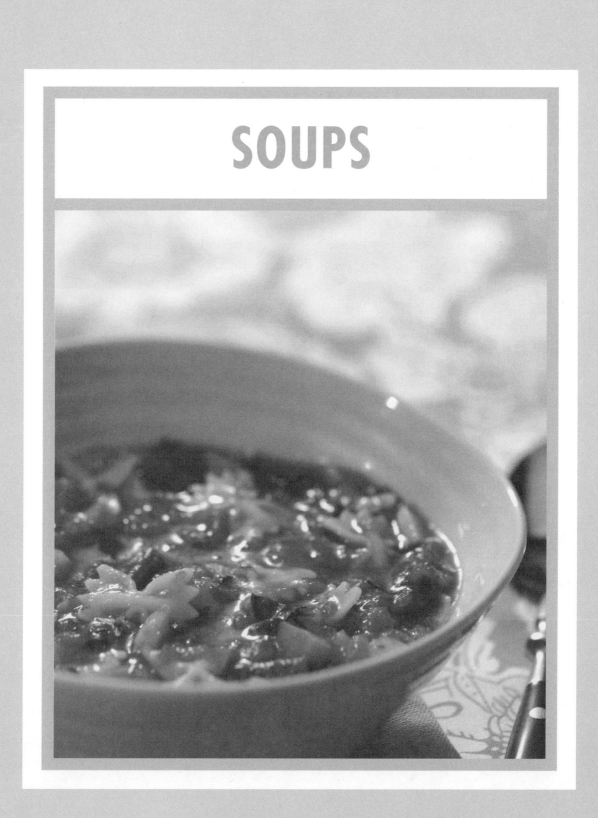

Broccoli Soup

SERVES 4

This is one of the easiest and best recipes to have in your repertoire since it involves so few ingredients and yet packs tons of flavor. The vibrant color makes it appealing to people of all ages. It is also simple to substitute other vegetables for the broccoli, making this an easy recipe to modify with whatever you have in the kitchen.

5 cups water

sea salt

1 head of broccoli, stem removed, cut into florets (about 2–3 cups)

1 tablespoon olive oil

3 cloves of garlic, peeled and slightly crushed

2 cups chicken or vegetable stock (or water)

¼ cup pine nuts

¼ cup fresh mint leaves

PREPARATION

Bring 5 cups water to a boil in a medium pot. Add a few pinches of salt to water and toss in broccoli. Cook for 30 seconds and drain immediately.

Heat oil in sauté pan over medium-high heat and add garlic; sauté 30–45 seconds, until fragrant. Add broccoli and sauté for 1 minute. Add stock and cook 1 more minute. Transfer entire pan's contents to a blender. Add pine nuts, mint, and a dash of salt. Blend until smooth* and taste for seasoning.

VARIATIONS

Substitute asparagus or cauliflower for the broccoli.

*When blending hot ingredients of any kind, either remove the lid and use a loose dish towel in its place, or remove the inner circular lid on blender, allowing steam to escape and preventing explosive buildup.

- Make extra garlic-broccoli sauté; it's a fantastic side dish for any poultry or meat dish.
- Freeze a portion of the soup and use it later as a light sauce for pasta or polenta, including Shepherd's Polenta (page 161) and Polenta "Lasagna" (page 162).

Raw Broccoli Soup

SERVES 4

This is a raw version of my Broccoli Soup. Refreshing and hearty, it is a perfect dish to accompany some rice and beans or pasta.

½ cup raw pine nuts, cashews, or almonds

1 head broccoli, cut into florets (about 2–3 cups)

1 clove garlic

1 tablespoon olive oil or coconut oil

3 cups water or vegetable stock

2 teaspoons raw honey

½ cup packed spinach leaves, washed and rinsed

¼ cup fresh mint leaves

¼ cup fresh parsley

sea salt

PREPARATION

This recipe is best prepared using a Vita-mix, but a good food processor will also yield excellent results.

Soak nuts in ½ cup water while preparing the rest of the soup.

Add garlic to the bowl of a food processor. Mince finely. Add soaked and drained nuts and oil, and pulse until smooth. Add 2½ cups water (or stock) and 1 cup of the broccoli; blend until smooth. Add the rest of the broccoli and remaining ingredients and pulse until smooth. Taste; adjust seasoning if needed. Serve at room temperature.

Miso Soup

Miso has long existed as a source of good health and longevity in Japan. Two of its greatest assets are its ability to remove heavy metals from the body and its ability to protect the body from the effects of radiation, properties that were first discovered after the atomic bombing of Nagasaki during World War II. Miso contains an alkaloid that binds heavy metals, such as radioactive strontium, and also contains an anti-cancer isoflavone called genistein.

The process of fermentation that creates miso can take years, and the paste can be prepared using soybeans, the classic preparation, or chickpeas, azuki beans, barley, brown rice, or any legume. Miso is a good source of micronutrients and some B vitamins. Since soybeans contain all essential amino acids, soybean miso is a complete protein. Miso also facilitates the body's absorption of calcium and magnesium, both of which are important to the athlete.

Keep in mind that you should not use any metallic utensils with miso paste—for cooking or for eating—as the miso will pick up the metallic flavor easily. Use wooden or ceramic forks and spoons instead.

2 cups chicken or vegetable stock, or water

1½ tablespoons miso

1 tablespoon tamari or soy sauce, such as Nama Shoyu

1 tablespoon mirin (sweet rice cooking wine)

¾ cup wakame (dried seaweed), soaked and drained, or ¼ cup plain or smoked dulse

2 tablespoons sliced scallions

1 teaspoon red pepper flakes (optional)

PREPARATION

In a small pot, bring stock almost to a boil. Place miso in serving bowl and pour ½ cup stock over it and let the miso dissolve. Add remaining stock and ingredients and stir to combine.

GOOD ACCOMPANIMENTS

- Soba noodles
- Pea sprouts or sunflower sprouts
- Frozen peas or corn during winter months
- Summer string beans, shell peas, or corn

VARIATION

Miso soup is a great way to easily bring leftovers together into a quick and nutritious meal. Most days I have extra soba noodles and/or roasted chicken in my fridge and the days that I have both I prepare some miso soup to bring them together.

As soon as I pour off some stock or liquid to dissolve my miso paste, I add my chicken and noodles to the remaining water. Once the miso has dissolved, add it to the rest of the liquid along with some fresh kale, spinach, or other green, and enjoy.

Easy Minestrone

This fall/winter soup is easy to prepare. You can vary the recipe according to what you have in your freezer or fridge. It's always satisfying and will warm you inside and out.

2–3 tablespoons olive oil

1 medium onion, chopped

1 large carrot, chopped

2 stalks celery, chopped

1 medium turnip, chopped

2 cloves garlic, chopped

1 large can whole peeled tomatoes

sea salt

2 cups chicken or vegetable stock (or water)

3 cups assorted fresh or frozen vegetables (such as corn, peas, green beans, broccoli, cauliflower)

1 tablespoon chopped fresh oregano (or 1 teaspoon dried)

1 tablespoon chopped fresh thyme (or 1 teaspoon dried)

1 tablespoon chopped fresh parsley

2 cups toasted buckwheat groats or other leftover grain or pasta, cooked

PREPARATION

Heat olive oil in medium-sized Dutch oven or large pot. Sauté chopped onion, carrot, celery, and turnip for 2–3 minutes. Add garlic and sauté 1 minute or until fragrant. Pour liquid from can of tomatoes into the pot, temporarily reserving the tomatoes. Pour the tomatoes into a bowl and crush them with your hands, then add to the pot. Season liberally with salt and taste for seasoning.

Add stock to pot and bring to a simmer. Add the remaining vegetables, herbs, and grain. Cook until vegetables are tender; time will vary depending upon the vegetables you have used.

SALADS

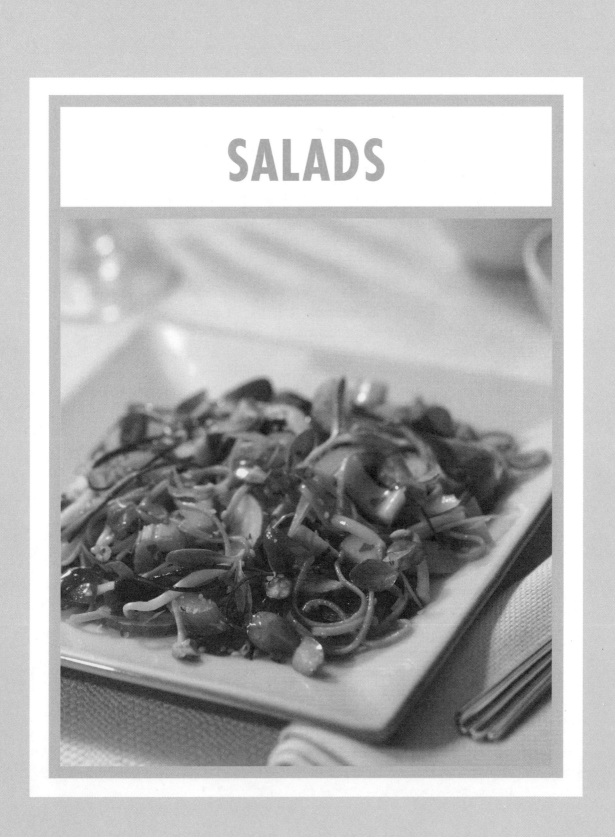

SALADS & DRESSINGS

A great chef I once worked for used to say it's all about the sauce. He understood the importance of fresh ingredients, but there is magic when a sauce is added that can really enhance a dish. Salad dressings are similar. They bring together and enhance all of the great components in a fresh, raw, or cooked salad. Dressings can be easy to prepare, and you can make plenty at one time. Quite often I will use a dressing I have in the fridge with a piece of fish or meat I just pulled off the grill.

The standard ratio of oil to vinegar for a classic dressing is 3:1 or 4:1. I enjoy a bit more acid or tang to my dressings, so I add more vinegar or citrus than the standard ratio. Salt is the ingredient that binds together the oil and vinegar. Black pepper can be added to your liking.

I like to depart from the standard vinegars and oils and use ones that have more beneficial health properties. I also avoid vinegars that are not raw, and I mainly use brown rice vinegar and apple cider vinegar due to their great health benefits as well as their flavor. It is also essential to choose oils that have been expeller- and/or cold-pressed, and are extra virgin. Heat-pressed oils have lost valuable nutrients and are subject to rancidity. "Extra-virgin" means that the oil was made from the first pressing of the fruit, seed, or nut. Polyunsaturated oils such as corn, canola, and safflower are also subject to rancidity, so I use a wide range of oils such as pumpkin seed, walnut, hemp seed, flax seed, sesame seed, olive, and almond.

Most of my salads are a combination of raw vegetables that are in season. For these salads, it's easiest to make the dressing right in the bowl along with vegetables. As I add each ingredient, I toss the vegetables lightly and taste each new layer as they blend together, adjusting for taste. Greens on their own are generally too delicate to withstand all of the stirring necessary to distribute the dressing evenly, so when eating greens only I like my dressings on the side.

Herb Salad with Tomatoes and Lemon–Olive Oil Dressing

SERVES 2

I had just made some pan-roasted chicken, and I needed a quick side dish that would be a fresh counterpart. I went to my herb garden and quickly grabbed the ingredients for what has come to be one of my favorite salads. It is a fantastic accompaniment for any weeknight meal since it's basically whatever herbs you have either in the fridge or, even better, the garden. Feel free to substitute herbs as needed or desired—the dressing is so versatile it's friendly to all sorts of mixtures.

2 tablespoons lime juice or lemon juice (about 1 lime or ¾ lemon)
1 tablespoon olive oil
sea salt
1 cup packed fresh parsley leaves
¼ cup fresh mint leaves
¼ cup fresh basil leaves (about 5–7 medium-sized leaves), torn into bite-sized pieces
½ cup halved cherry tomatoes

PREPARATION

Whisk juice, oil, and salt in a small bowl. Toss remaining ingredients with dressing and serve immediately.

GOOD ACCOMPANIMENTS

- Pan-Roasted Chicken (page 221)
- Whole Baked Fish (page 203)
- Sandwiches
- Quinoa Tabouleh (page 178)
- Falafel

Asian Chopped Chicken in Lettuce Cups

SERVES 3–4

These simple "cups" are always a crowd pleaser and make a great appetizer or light lunch when throwing a party. Refreshing and light, the combination of textures and flavors makes this dish a hard one to beat.

1 head fresh buttercup or red Boston lettuce

2 tablespoons fish sauce

3 tablespoons Nama Shoyu or low-sodium soy sauce

1 tablespoon raw honey

1¼ teaspoons red pepper flakes

1 tablespoon toasted sesame oil

1 tablespoon olive oil

1 tablespoon minced garlic

1 tablespoon minced fresh gingerroot

1 pound (about 3–4 portions) boneless, skinless chicken breast, finely chopped

sea salt

1 large carrot, julienned

1 medium cucumber, peeled, seeded, and julienned

1 cup pea shoot sprouts

¼ cup chopped scallions

½ cup sunflower seeds, pine nuts, or chopped cashews

PREPARATION

Pull all leaves from the head of lettuce, leaving the smaller core leaves attached to the stem; keep for later use. Thoroughly wash the leaves and run through a salad spinner or pat dry with a cloth.

In a small bowl, whisk together fish sauce, Nama Shoyu, honey, and red pepper flakes.

Heat a sauté pan over medium-high heat. Add sesame and olive oils and let warm for 30 seconds (do not overheat or the garlic will burn when it hits the pan). Add the garlic and ginger. Sauté for 30 seconds, then add chicken and a pinch of salt. Cook chicken 3–5 minutes or until completely cooked through. Add the sauce mixture to the pan. Cook until sauce reduces by half (about 5 minutes) and remove the pan from the heat.

Arrange lettuce leaves on a platter or individual plates and sprinkle a few pieces of carrot, cucumber, pea shoots or other sprouts, and scallions into each "cup." Top with chicken and a few seeds or nuts.

GOOD ACCOMPANIMENTS

- Brown rice (page 183)
- Quinoa (page 174)
- Soba noodles dressed with a bit of hempseed oil

Daily Antipasto

SERVES 4–6

This is one of the best ways to use extra or leftover vegetables in your fridge and can be made with whatever is in season. It's perfect as a quick snack as well as a side dish for something coming off the grill. Stored in an airtight mason jar, it will keep for a few weeks and get better and better, both in flavor and nutrient content, as it marinates.

sea salt

2 cups broccoli florets plus the broccoli stem, peeled and cut into chunks*

2 cups cauliflower florets

2–3 large carrots, peeled and cut into chunks

2–3 celery stalks, cut into chunks

1 jar marinated artichoke hearts, cut into chunks

1 yellow pepper, seeded, cut into chunks

1 red pepper, seeded, cut into chunks

1 large cucumber, peeled, seeded, and cut into chunks

1 cup halved cherry tomatoes

1 small shallot, diced

¼ cup chopped fresh parsley

2 tablespoons sesame seeds

3 tablespoons hempseed oil

½ cup raw apple cider vinegar**

* I like to use the entirety of my ingredients when possible, and broccoli stem has a great texture and a subtle flavor. Peel the tough outer skin of the stem, revealing the whitish core, and cut into chunks. No need to blanch with the florets; use the stem raw.

** Raw apple cider vinegar, which has a sweet, slightly caramel flavor, is full of active enzymes and prebiotics. It increases the microflora of your inner ecosystem and strengthens your immune system, a boon for athletes who constantly tax their immune system by increasing their cortisol levels with the stresses of training. It also aids in digestion and helps alkalize the body's blood. (Most Americans have an acidic blood pH, which can lead to joint and muscle problems as well as difficulty in processing free radicals that accumulate due to oxidation during exercise.)

PREPARATION

Bring 4–5 quarts of water to a boil and add 2 tablespoons salt to the water. Prepare a bowl of ice water (preferably in the sink next to where you will drain the broccoli). Boil the broccoli florets and cauliflower for 30–45 seconds, until just barely cooked. The broccoli will turn a vibrant green color. Remove, drain, and immediately plunge into the ice water to cool. This method of blanching and shocking keeps the broccoli and cauliflower crisp and retains the broccoli's bright green color.

Add broccoli and cauliflower florets to a large bowl and add the remaining ingredients. Toss until very well combined and then either portion out as a side dish or put into mason jars for longer-term storage.

Marinated Beet Salad with Sugar Snap Peas and Cabbage Slaw

SERVES 4

Beets are generally eaten cooked, but this is a great way to eat them raw after marinating them in apple cider vinegar. They retain their beautiful color, their sweetness, and all of their great nutrients. This salad blends texture, flavor, appearance, and nutrients, and it gets better with time when kept in the fridge.

2 cups red or golden beets, peeled and thinly sliced

1 small head green cabbage, shredded

2 tablespoons raw apple cider vinegar, divided

1 medium cucumber, peeled, seeded, and cut into small chunks

1¼ cups fresh sugar snap peas or 1 cup fresh peas from the pod

sea salt

Dressing

¼ cup olive oil

¼ cup toasted sesame oil

1 tablespoon brown rice vinegar

3 tablespoons raw apple cider vinegar

1 tablespoon black sesame seeds or hemp seeds

1 tablespoon chopped fresh mint

1 tablespoon grated lime zest

sea salt

PREPARATION

Before preparing the rest of the salad, toss sliced beets with 1 tablespoon of the apple cider vinegar and a pinch of salt. Turn every 15–20 minutes while preparing the rest of the ingredients.

Shred cabbage. In a separate bowl, combine cabbage with a pinch of salt and the remaining tablespoon of the apple cider vinegar. Toss every 3–5 minutes, draining released water each time, for about 20 minutes total.

Drain the bowls of beets and cabbage. Portion the cabbage onto 4 plates.

Using the bowl the cabbage was in, whisk all the dressing ingredients together. Add the beets, cucumber, and peas, and combine. Portion one-fourth of the salad on top of each plate of cabbage; serve.

GOOD ADDITIONS

- Grilled or roasted chicken
- Cooked or sprouted chickpeas

How to use a mandoline

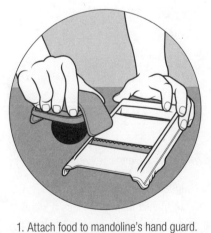

1. Attach food to mandoline's hand guard.

2. Tilt mandoline on an angle.
Apply gentle pressure and slide food down, against the blade.

Roasted Beet Salad

SERVES 4

Beets are great hot or cold, and this salad can be served either way. Their sweetness marries well with tang of acidity, which makes citrus an excellent counterpart. I love to make a dressing with lime and orange, but the nuttiness of apple cider vinegar is a great option.

Beets

3 cups beets, cut into small chunks

2 tablespoons olive oil or coconut oil

3 cloves garlic, peeled

1 sprig fresh rosemary or ½ tablespoon dried rosemary

sea salt

Dressing

2 tablespoons hempseed oil

1 tablespoon lemon or lime zest

2 tablespoons fresh lime, lemon, or orange juice, or apple cider vinegar

1 tablespoon hemp seeds, sesame seeds, or sunflower seeds

¼ cup chopped almonds (optional)

1 tablespoon chopped fresh parsley

1 tablespoon chopped fresh mint

sea salt

PREPARATION

Preheat oven to 425 degrees.

In a small mixing bowl, toss the chopped beets with olive oil, garlic, rosemary, and salt.

Beets cook best with some steam involved, so I suggest cooking them in pouches. Cut a large piece of aluminum foil approximately 12–14 inches in length. Place a sheet of parchment paper slightly smaller than the foil on top. Lay out the beets on half of the parchment, and fold over both the parchment and the foil. Crimp up the sides into a tight pouch.

Place on baking sheet and bake 35–40 minutes, or until beets are fork-tender.

While the beets cook, whisk together all ingredients for dressing in a separate bowl. Adjust salt to taste.

Once the beets are done, slowly open pouch (be careful of hot steam) and let cool 5 minutes. Transfer to a bowl and toss with dressing.

The Essential Salad

SERVES 4

One of the most common issues I find with individuals living active life-styles is a deficiency of micronutrients, which can lead to injury. This salad, which incorporates the seaweeds arame and wakame, is not only full of flavor and variety but also contains the essential micronutrients and minerals that the active body requires. It is great on its own or as a side dish to almost any protein.

Salad

1 cup arame, soaked and drained

1 cup wakame, soaked and drained

1 cup soba noodles or rice noodles (optional)

1 cucumber, peeled and diced

3 stalks celery, chopped, and inner leaves (optional)

2 carrots, peeled and sliced

1 yellow pepper, seeded, cut into strips

½ cup radishes, sliced

1 cup mung bean sprouts

1 cup snow pea sprouts or sunflower sprouts

¼ cup hulled hemp seeds

1 teaspoon red pepper flakes (optional)

Dressing

1 tablespoon minced fresh gingerroot

3 tablespoons Nama Shoyu or tamari

3 tablespoons mirin (sweet rice wine for cooking)

2 tablespoons brown rice vinegar or apple cider vinegar

2 tablespoons sesame oil

Soak arame and wakame according to package instructions and drain well. Squeeze with hands if necessary to remove excess water. If using soba or rice noodles, prepare according to package instructions and drain.

While seaweeds are soaking (about 10–15 minutes), assemble rest of salad ingredients in a large bowl.

Whisk dressing ingredients in a medium-sized bowl. Combine dressing with drained seaweeds, noodles, and remaining salad ingredients. Toss well and serve.

Black Lentil Salad

SERVES 2

You can double this recipe and reserve the extra to make Lentil Burgers; see recipe on page 180.

1 cup black lentils
1 carrot, diced
2 stalks celery, diced
3 tablespoons diced shallots
3 tablespoons hempseed oil or walnut oil
¼ cup chopped fresh parsley
1 tablespoon raw apple cider vinegar
sea salt

PREPARATION

Rinse lentils and sort through, removing unwanted material or debris. Place lentils in small pot and cover with 3 inches of water. Bring lentils to a boil, reduce heat, and simmer for about 30 minutes or until lentils are tender but not mushy. When done, remove from heat and pour off remaining liquid. Set aside to cool. Once cooled, add remaining ingredients and toss together.

GOOD ADDITIONS

- In-season vegetables like sweet peppers, tomatoes, cucumbers, radishes, etc.
- Almonds, pumpkin seeds, or sunflower seeds.

DRESSINGS, DIPS & TOPPINGS

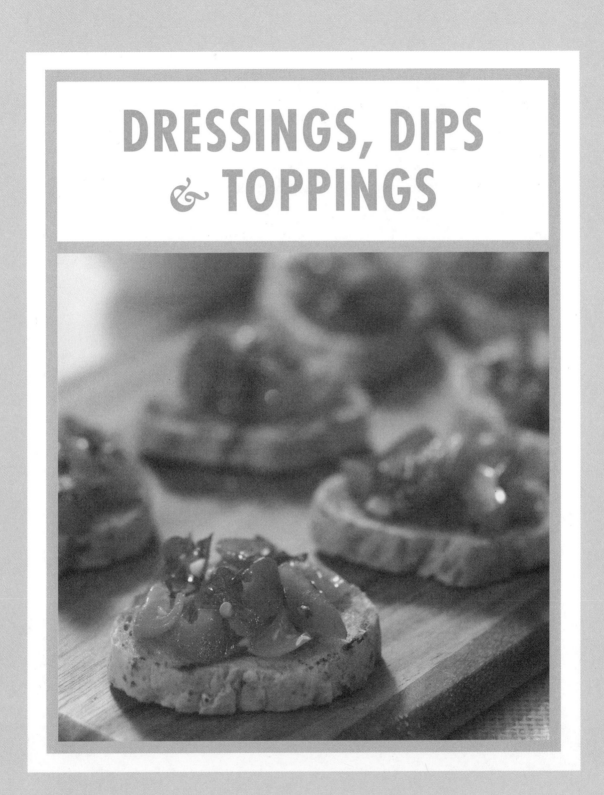

Lemon Tahini Dressing

MAKES 1½ CUPS

This is a salad dressing that can also be used to add flavor to other dishes; see "Good Accompaniments" for suggestions.

¾ cup raw sesame tahini
¼ cup olive oil
2 tablespoons hempseed oil
½ cup fresh lemon juice (about 4 lemons)
1 tablespoon raw honey
1 clove garlic, minced
1 tablespoon raw apple cider vinegar
1 tablespoon chopped fresh parsley
sea salt

PREPARATION

Mix all ingredients in blender or the bowl of a food processor, or whisk together vigorously in a small mixing bowl. Refrigerate in an airtight container for up to 1 week.

GOOD ACCOMPANIMENTS

- Hearty lettuce (kale or romaine)
- Grilled chicken or fish
- Turkey Burgers (page 226)

Ginger Miso Dressing

MAKES 1 CUP

I use this dressing most often on Asian baby salad greens such as bok choy, tatsoi, and mizuna with raw vegetables and bamboo shoots, but it is also great with grilled mushrooms and steamed vegetables.

½ cup olive oil

¼ cup hempseed oil or sesame oil

⅓ cup raw apple cider vinegar or rice wine vinegar

1 tablespoon miso paste

1 tablespoon chopped shallot

½ tablespoon chopped fresh gingerroot

1 tablespoon chopped fresh parsley

1 tablespoon raw honey (optional)

sea salt

PREPARATION

Add all ingredients to large bowl and whisk together. Keeps in airtight container up to 1 week in refrigerator.

Sesame Citrus Dressing

MAKES 1 CUP

I use this dressing for salads as well as grilled chicken and fish.

¼ cup olive oil
¼ cup flaxseed oil
¼ cup sesame oil or toasted sesame oil
2 tablespoons brown rice vinegar
3 tablespoons fresh lime juice
1 tablespoon minced shallot
1 teaspoon black sesame seeds
1 teaspoon hemp seeds
1 tablespoon chopped fresh parsley
1 tablespoon chopped mint (optional)
1 tablespoon chopped cilantro (optional)
sea salt to taste

PREPARATION

Add all ingredients to bowl and whisk together until combined.

Sundried Tomato Spread

MAKES ABOUT 1 CUP

I always have this in my fridge. It is super-easy to make and goes well with sandwiches of turkey and hummus, or chicken salad, or as a condiment for beef. Try to find tomatoes that have some pliability; look for them in the bulk foods aisle, or find them packaged (for this recipe, the ones packed in oil are less desirable; if you must use them, you will need to reduce the amount of oil in the recipe, probably by half).

1½ cups sundried tomatoes, not packed in oil
½ cup olive oil
2 cloves garlic
2 tablespoons chopped fresh parsley
2 tablespoons chopped fresh mint
1 tablespoon chopped fresh oregano or 1 teaspoon dried oregano
¼ cup pine nuts
sea salt

PREPARATION

If the tomatoes are really dry, soak them in just a bit of warm water while gathering the rest of the ingredients. If they are soft, add them straight into the food processor with olive oil. Add the rest of the ingredients and process to an almost smooth texture. Transfer to a jar or other container and refrigerate. Keeps up to a month.

Consistency will vary, so you may need to add more oil to get the texture you like. My preference is to have it wet enough to spread easily, but not to the point where it is sitting in oil.

VARIATION

Use roasted red peppers instead of sundried tomatoes, or add some to the recipe mix above.

Goat Cheese Spreads

MAKES ABOUT 1 CUP EACH

Fresh raw goat cheese is the "cream cheese" of my home. Raw milk contains protein, fats, and enzymes that are great for an athlete's diet. The shelf life of this spread is not as great as that of tahini, but it is so delicious that it won't be around long anyway.

Base for each recipe
8 ounces fresh raw goat cheese (also known as chèvre)

PREPARATION

Slightly sweet
Add 1 tablespoon raw honey and 1 tablespoon chopped fresh mint leaves. Stir or whip until combined and serve with strawberries, apples, or pears.

Savory
Add 2 tablespoons chopped fresh rosemary and 1 tablespoon chopped fresh parsley, sea salt, and freshly ground black pepper. Stir or whip until combined and serve as a condiment for grilled or roasted meats.

Spicy
Add a few chopped chipotle peppers or other hot peppers and a dash of cayenne. Stir or whip until combined and use as a spicy spread for tortilla-based sandwiches or snacks.

GOOD ACCOMPANIMENTS

- Sandwiches (my favorite is sprouted bread, sliced avocado, sunflower sprouts, and a tomato with the spicy spread)
- Raw veggies
- Sprouted breads or tortillas

Smoked Bluefish and Goat Cheese

SERVES 2

Some people are turned off by the strong smell and oil content of blue-fish, but the oil is what makes it a healthy choice. In fact, bluefish has almost as many EFAs as salmon. The oil content makes it an excellent choice for smoking or grilling. To save preparation time, this recipe uses pre-smoked bluefish.

8 ounces smoked bluefish fillet
8 ounces (1 cup) fresh raw goat cheese
1 teaspoon olive oil
1 tablespoon chopped fresh chives
1 tablespoon chopped fresh parsley

PREPARATION

In a small mixing bowl, break the bluefish apart with a fork. Add the goat cheese and continue to mash, blending the two together. Add oil as needed to help loosen the mixture. Keep working until well incorporated and almost of a soft and fluffy texture. Add chives and parsley and mix.

GOOD ACCOMPANIMENTS

- Sandwiches
- Soft-boiled eggs
- Polenta

VARIATIONS

Try other herbs, such as sage, cilantro, dill, and basil, according to preference.

Bruschetta Topping

SERVES 4

Bruschetta is a perfect food that guarantees a smile every time. The contrast in texture between the crunchy grilled bread and the soft, sweet tomatoes is a full-body experience and makes this a light, healthy, and satisfying snack.

1 pound fresh Roma tomatoes (about 4–5), diced

3 tablespoons olive oil, plus more for brushing

sea salt

2–3 garlic cloves, minced

1 tablespoon chopped fresh oregano

1 tablespoon chopped fresh thyme

2 teaspoons crushed red pepper flakes

1 tablespoon chopped fresh parsley

5 fresh basil leaves, chopped

½ whole-grain baguette, cut into 1-inch slices

PREPARATION

An important part of making this dish is to taste as you add each new ingredient. Adjust the seasoning and quantities as you go (it's good to have a little extra of each ingredient on hand, if possible).

Start by placing the tomatoes, 3 tablespoons olive oil, and salt in a bowl. Toss together. Add the garlic and mix. Add oregano and mix. Add thyme and mix. Add red pepper and mix. Add parsley and mix. Add basil and mix.

Let sit at room temperature for at least 1 hour before using.

Brush the baguette slices with olive oil and either grill or broil in the oven. Top with tomato mixture and enjoy.

VARIATION

You can use this as a "pizza sauce" by topping a sprouted tortilla with a few tablespoons of the tomato mixture and then sprinkling some raw grated cheese on top. Pop the entire thing in the oven for a few minutes, until the cheese has melted and the sauce has warmed through.

This topping can also be used on grilled fish or meat. Not only does it satisfy the "cooked foods/raw foods" rule, but it also adds a great contrast of texture and temperature.

Guacamole

SERVES 2–3

Avocados are one of the most athlete-friendly foods out there. Packed with tons of vitamins, nutrients, and good fats, they should be in everyone's kitchen when available. Always be sure the avocado is ripe (semisoft to the touch and bright green on the inside), and don't worry about it browning—acid is what keeps an avocado's color bright green, so the lime juice in this recipe will do the trick. If you are using only half an avocado and want to keep the other half fresh, lightly squeeze a lemon or lime over it before putting it in the fridge. If you want to prepare this ahead of time, the trick is to leave the seed within the mixture and cover very tightly. Guacamole is typically eaten with tortilla chips, but I also like it as a spread for sandwiches, a side for grilled meats, and an accompaniment to just about anything else I can think of!

1 large ripe avocado
1 clove garlic, minced
sea salt
juice of ½ lime
2–3 tablespoons hempseed oil or olive oil

PREPARATION

Opening an avocado is intimidating to many, but the correct method is easy. Using a sharp knife, split the avocado lengthwise and twist apart. Place a folded dish towel in your nondominant hand, and then place the half of the avocado with the pit on top of the dish towel. Bring the knife down into the pit with gentle but firm force (don't be afraid—that's what the dish towel is there for). Twist the knife until the pit pops out attached to the knife, and then use the dish towel to remove the pit from the blade. Discard. Scoop the flesh into a small mixing bowl.

Using a fork, mash the avocado. Add the garlic, a bit of salt, and lime juice. Mash again, then add oil and more salt, taste, and continue to mash and add oil until desired texture is reached.

How to remove an avocado pit

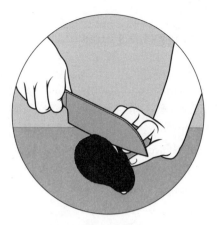

1. Slice lengthwise.

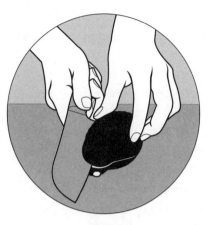

2. Run knife all the way around.

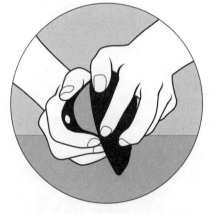

3. Twist halves in opposite directions, exposing seed.

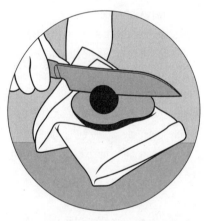

4. With a dish towel, hold seed half in one hand and bring knife firmly down onto seed. Twist seed and lift out.

Fresh Salsas

EACH RECIPE MAKES APPROXIMATELY 3 CUPS

The word *salsa* means "sauce" in Spanish, and there are many different varieties depending upon geographic location. For me, it varies depending upon the time of the year and the availability of vegetables, but is always built upon a foundation of fresh tomatoes. If I can't find fresh, local tomatoes, then you won't find salsa in my fridge. It begins when the first cherry tomatoes are ready, progresses through the summer heirlooms, and finishes off with the tomatillos of fall.

Mild

1 pint cherry tomatoes, halved

2 tablespoons chopped fresh parsley

1 tablespoon chopped fresh mint (or 1 teaspoon dried)

1 clove garlic, minced

2 tablespoons diced shallot or ¼ cup diced red onion

2 tablespoons hempseed oil or olive oil

1 tablespoon raw apple cider vinegar

2 tablespoons lime juice

sea salt

Spicy

1 pound fresh Roma tomatoes (about 5–7), diced

2 cloves garlic, minced

½ medium-sized red onion, finely diced

1–5 chili peppers (jalapeño, serrano, habanera, or bird), according to your heat preference

2 tablespoons chopped fresh cilantro

1 tablespoon chopped fresh parsley

½ tablespoon chopped fresh oregano (optional)

1 tablespoon hempseed oil

juice of 1 lime

sea salt

For each salsa, simply combine all ingredients in a mixing bowl and stir together. It's best to let it sit at room temperature for at least an hour so the flavors can blend before serving.

Grilled Tomato and Jalapeño Salsa

MAKES ABOUT 1½ CUPS

This is the perfect accompaniment to any summer grilled meal or a great appetizer to serve at a party. If you have a multitiered gas grill, you can easily do this on the side as you prepare everything else. Or, for even deeper flavor, prepare on a charcoal grill.

2 medium-sized slicing tomatoes, cores removed (e.g., Beefsteak, Cherokee, Bradley, or Brandywine)
2 fresh jalapeño peppers
½ head of garlic, with skin on
2 tablespoons olive oil
sea salt
1 small white onion, trimmed and peeled
½ bunch fresh cilantro leaves (about 1 loosely packed cup)
juice of 1 lime

PREPARATION

Bring grill to high heat, so that you can hold your hand 3 inches above the grate for 3 seconds.

In a large mixing bowl, toss whole tomatoes, jalapeños, and garlic with olive oil and a pinch of salt. Coat evenly and place on grill. Cook until everything is slightly charred and softened, about 10–15 minutes, turning often.

Once cooked, place tomatoes and jalapeños in the bowl of a food processor or blender. Cut onion in half and add to food processor. Remove garlic cloves (they should squeeze out of their skins) and add to food processor, along with cilantro. Pulse until everything is well blended and of the texture of your choice—chunky or soupy. Taste for seasoning and stir in lime juice and salt as needed.

GOOD ACCOMPANIMENTS

- Braised Pork Chops (page 232)
- Beans and Brown Rice (page 182)
- Flank steak

Roasted Tomatillo Salsa

MAKES ABOUT 2 CUPS

1 pound fresh tomatillos, husks removed (roughly 12–16)

1 tablespoon olive oil

sea salt

¼ cup fresh cilantro leaves

1–2 chili peppers (jalapeño, serrano, bird)

2 cloves garlic

1 tablespoon hempseed oil

½ tablespoon raw honey

2 tablespoons fresh lime juice

½ onion, finely chopped

PREPARATION

Preheat oven to 450 degrees.

Rinse and dry tomatillos. Toss with oil and a pinch of salt. Place on baking sheet lined with parchment paper and roast for 5–7 minutes, until tomatillos are just wilting and slightly brown.

Remove from oven and place in blender or food processor with all of their juices. Blend with cilantro leaves, garlic, peppers, oil, honey, lime juice, and salt. Once it is broken down to a sauce, add onions and pulse a few times. Store in an airtight container in the fridge for up to 1 week.

VARIATION

Grill the tomatillos for a charred, smoky flavor instead of roasting them.

Raw Sauerkraut

Sauerkraut is a condiment, of course, but I also think of it as a snack, as I do other fermented foods such as kimchi, pickles, and cured olives. Making raw sauerkraut is simple; it's mostly about letting nature do the work. All you need do is assemble the ingredients and place them in the proper environment, at which point a process called lacto-fermentation takes over. Natural and healthy bacteria operate in three different stages and create an unfavorable environment to harmful bacteria, preserving the food while developing highly absorbable nutrients that are of great benefit to the athlete.

The health benefits of the fermentation process have been known for centuries. In his book *The Permaculture Book of Ferment and Human Nutrition,* Bill Mollison identifies fermented foods—fruit, vegetables, fish, and dairy products—that are found around the globe. These foods boost the immune system, helping to prevent common colds and flu, and aid in the recovery of a physically stressed body. Fermented foods are known to be a great digestive as well; as Mollison describes, they are "pre-digested" and therefore capable of providing the intestinal tract with healthy bacteria along with easily assimilated nutrients. These "good" bacteria will also help fight harmful ones like *E. coli* and salmonella. In addition, they fight the overgrowth of unhealthy yeasts that lead to conditions such as joint and muscle pains and candida.

Fermented foods contain high amounts of antioxidants that will collect the free radicals produced during exercise. They help to facilitate the breakdown and assimilation of proteins as well as the breakdown of antinutrients such as phytic acid, found in all grains.

I believe these foods are an essential part of an athletic diet, and I recommend that you eat something raw and/or fermented with every meal.

When I make sauerkraut, I always make a big batch—about three gallons. Stored in a cool, dry place like a basement or fridge, it can last months. It's one of those things that I never have around long enough to find out when it does spoil, but I have eaten mine after three months and found that the flavor only gets better. In fact, Captain James Cook, the legendary explorer and voyager, always had sauerkraut on his ship—the high vitamin C content helped prevent scurvy—and some of his trips lasted more than two years.

You can ferment sauerkraut in any clean glass jar; I use a 1-gallon jar. Sauerkraut fermenting crocks also can be used; of these, I have found the Harsch crocks to be the best.

There are many variations that you can make to this basic recipe using herbs, spices, and other vegetables, so be creative.

5–10 pounds green cabbage, depending on size of container
3–7 tablespoons sea salt

PREPARATION

Shred cabbage into thin slices using a knife, mandoline, or other tool. I simply use a knife, cutting the head in half and then slicing the cabbage lengthwise. When I get to the core, I turn the cabbage on the cut edge and then slice down the back and around the core on either side. You can also just slice right through to the base including the core, but I tend not to. Place the shredded cabbage in a large mixing bowl, sprinkle on a bit of salt (slightly less than ½ tablespoon per pound), and toss.

Place a handful or so of the cabbage into the fermenting container and tamp it down using a wooden spoon, mallet, or other utensil until it is tightly packed. Add any extracted water from the mixing bowl. Continue this process until you have transferred all of the cabbage to the container.

Once all of the cabbage has been packed in, it needs a weight to stay submerged. When I use a 1-gallon jar, I fill a mason jar with water, place it on top of the cabbage, and then cover everything with a cheesecloth or kitchen towel. For larger jars, I put a few intact cabbage leaves over the shredded ones, followed by a plate and then a suitable weight. Do not cover the jar with a tight-fitting lid at this point; allow some exposure to the air.

Over the course of the first 24 hours, the water from the cabbage will continue to be extracted and will eventually rise above the cabbage itself with the help of your weight. If this does not happen, you will need to prepare some saltwater (1 tablespoon salt to 1 cup of water) and pour it on top of the cabbage until it is covered by an inch.

Place the container out of the way, ideally where the temperature is around 72–75 degrees, and let the process begin. After 5–7 days, you can begin to taste the kraut for its tangy flavor. During this time you might notice a whitish bloom on the surface of the water covering the cabbage. Simply remove it with a spoon; it will not affect your kraut.

After approximately 2 weeks, depending on the temperature and amount of salt used, you can cover the container with a tight-fitting lid and place it in the fridge or in a cool spot in your basement. (The more salt you use, the slower the fermentation; the warmer the temperature, the faster the fermentation.) Once stored, the fermentation will continue to proceed but at a much slower rate, and the flavor will become more tangy.

When the sauerkraut has reached its full flavor, fill a large mason jar from the main container to use in the kitchen, and leave the rest in the basement. Be sure the remaining cabbage is packed down tightly so that it is covered by water whenever you are storing it outside of the fridge. Add more salted water to keep it covered if need be.

VARIATIONS

- Use red cabbage instead of green, or use a mix of both.
- Add some julienned carrots, chopped fresh gingerroot, and red pepper flakes.
- Use Chinese cabbage along with julienned carrots, scallions, gingerroot, garlic, and red pepper flakes to make kimchi.
- Add caraway or mustard seeds and/or some herbs such as thyme, oregano, and dill.

Brined Vegetables

This is another way of fermenting foods such as cucumbers for pickles, and it's a great way to store vegetables for other seasons.

PREPARATION

Clean the vegetables or fruit that you would like to ferment: cucumbers, radishes, beets, garlic, and tomatoes are good candidates. Scrub the skin well with a brush under running water. The amount you prepare will depend on the sizes of the vegetables and container you use. You want to pack the contents in as tightly as possible (quartering or slicing beets and larger items might be helpful). Weight the contents as for sauerkraut. Dissolve 2 tablespoons of sea salt per 1 quart of water. Add this brine to cover the contents by at least 2 inches. Follow the remainder of the instructions for making sauerkraut.

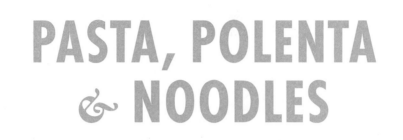

PASTA, POLENTA & NOODLES

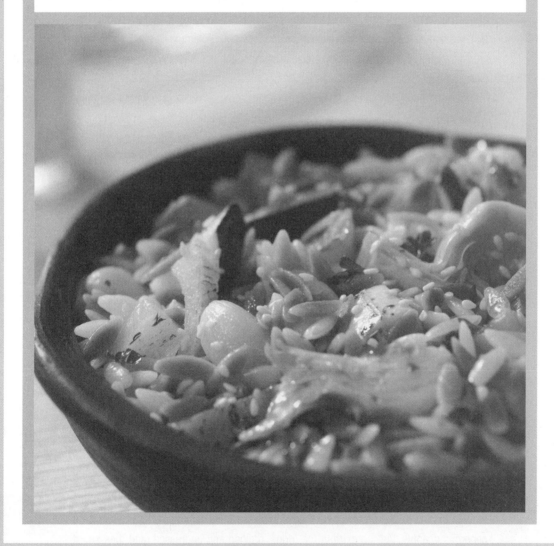

PASTA

I don't know about you, but in my world pasta is king. As much as I love and value whole grains, pasta, to me, is the food of the soul. Although I could eat it almost every day, I try to restrain myself, so it becomes even more special when I do indulge. In fact, sometimes I feel as though the only reason I exercise is so that I can eat what I want—and pasta is always number one on the list!

I was fortunate to spend a portion of my culinary career working in what I still think is one of the best Italian restaurants in the country. It was a tiny place in Fort Collins, Colorado (of all places), called Pulcinella Ristorante. I was often assigned to the grill, and one of the chefs would chastise me regularly for taking my eyes off the fire to watch the pasta preparations. To this day I continue to prepare some of the same dishes that my wandering eyes took in—my versions of them, anyway. As simple as some of those dishes were in their culinary perfection, they did not always fit into a busy work and training schedule, so I had to come up with some quick and easy ways to prepare my favorite food. I'll share some with you!

First and foremost, you must choose high-quality pasta. Cheap pasta is a disaster. I have yet to find a U.S.-based company that produces a good-quality, Old World–style, die-cast dry pasta made from durum semolina flour, so instead I look for organic fresh pasta produced locally. When I can't find that, I break down and purchase a packaged version that has been imported from Italy. I know this breaks my "buy local" credo, but in this case it's worth it.

Today you can also find pastas that are made with whole wheat, artichoke, spinach, spelt, quinoa, kamut, and vegetable flours. These can be great for cold pasta salads, but I find they tend to become a little gummy when prepared for hot dishes. When I am looking for a whole-grain noodle, I turn to the buckwheat, spelt, and kamut versions of soba or udon noodles.

Pasta definitely fits the "never prepare one meal at a time" idea. It takes the same amount of time to prepare a box as it does to prepare one serving, so I always make a generous quantity. Put the extra in the fridge, drained and undressed, and then add it later to chicken and greens for a salad; dress it with some sundried tomato spread or quick, fresh pesto; or reheat it at the last moment by draining your blanching water for broccoli over it and make it a side dish for almost any of the recipes in this book. You get the idea.

I also find it important to cook pasta in water that has been well salted, to the point where you can taste the salt if you dip your finger into the water and lick it. Most pasta directions call for 4–6 quarts of water per pound, but in my experience this amount takes too much time to boil and wastes too much energy. I cook smaller cuts of pasta (penne, for example) in a small pot filled with perhaps 2 quarts of water. The pasta cooks more quickly, and it never gets too gummy or starchy for my liking—as long as I am using good pasta.

Pasta should be removed from the heat when it is almost done so that you can finish the cooking in the saucepan. The starch helps to build the sauce structure and gives pasta its perfect al dente bite. If you are using a packaged pasta, I advise pulling it off the heat 1–2 minutes before the suggested cooking time on the box.

Linguine with Clams, Mint, and Tomatoes

SERVES 2

I think clams contain the essence of the sea. The liquid in the shell is ocean nectar, with a perfect balance of salty freshness. I love to eat clams raw at sundown with a cold beer, sharing adventure stories with friends. However, clams are best when the ocean waters are cool; as a reminder of their season, they should be eaten during months that have the letter "R" in them.

½ pound pasta of your choice (linguine is my favorite; penne works well too)
sea salt
2 tablespoons olive oil
3 cloves garlic, sliced
18 fresh clams in their shells, rinsed
red pepper flakes
¼ cup water
1 cup halved cherry tomatoes
2 tablespoons chopped fresh mint

PREPARATION

Bring water to boil, salt well, and add pasta. Cook according to package directions.

While the pasta cooks, heat olive oil in a pan with a tight-fitting lid over medium-high heat. Add garlic and cook for 30 seconds, until fragrant. Add clams and stir for 30 seconds. Add crushed red pepper and stir for 30 seconds. Then add water and cover tightly with lid.

The clams will start to pop open in about 5–7 minutes. Remove the clams as they open, place them on a plate, and then remove the pan from the heat.

Drain the pasta, reserving ½ cup of the pasta water. Return the pasta to the pot and add the clams with their juices. Add the tomatoes and mint and toss together, adding pasta water to loosen sauce if necessary. Serve immediately.

If tomatoes aren't in season, cut broccoli into florets to measure 2 cups and add to the pasta water 30 seconds before draining. Cook, drain, and toss with ingredients in place of tomatoes.

Pasta with Fresh
Roma Tomato Sauce and
Meat (Turkey or Beef),
Shrimp, or Scallops

SERVES 2

For those interested in a quick, fresh sauce, this dish can be prepared without meat to save prep time; see the variation at the recipe's end.

½ pound pasta of your choice

1 tablespoon olive oil

¾ pound ground beef or turkey, whole shrimp, or sea scallops (optional)

sea salt

1–2 garlic cloves, minced or sliced

1 pound fresh Roma tomatoes (about 4–5), diced

red pepper flakes

1 tablespoon chopped fresh parsley or basil

1–2 tablespoons grated raw cheese

PREPARATION

Bring water to boil and cook pasta according to package directions.

Heat olive oil in pan over medium-high heat for 1 minute. If using ground meat, add to pan with a pinch of salt and brown for 5 minutes, breaking up meat with a wooden spoon or fork. Drain all but 2 tablespoons of fat from pan.

Add garlic to pan and sauté 30 seconds, until fragrant. Add tomatoes and another pinch of salt. If using shrimp or scallops, add with tomatoes. Sauté 3–5 minutes.

By this time, the pasta should be done. Drain and reserve ¼ cup of the pasta water. Add pasta to pan along with crushed red pepper and toss together over heat for 1–2 minutes. If sauce is too dry, add a bit of pasta water.

Top with parsley or basil and cheese. Serve immediately.

VARIATION

To make a vegetarian version, wait 5 minutes into pasta cooking time before starting the sauce. Heat oil in pan. Add garlic and sauté 30 seconds, until fragrant. Add tomatoes and another pinch of salt. Sauté 3–5 minutes.

Tricolored Orzo with Grilled Vegetables

SERVES 2

I love having this pasta salad in my fridge because it is great after a solid physical outing. You can top it with leftover chicken or pork, have it alongside some hummus, make it a side dish to a turkey burger, grill up some shrimp or seared tuna, or just eat it by itself.

8 ounces tricolored (vegetable) orzo (or substitute regular orzo)

2 tablespoons hempseed oil

1 medium zucchini

1 bell pepper

1 fennel bulb

1 Japanese eggplant

1 garlic bulb

8 ounces (1 cup) marinated artichoke hearts

2 tablespoons chopped fresh parsley

2 tablespoons sesame seeds

½ bunch arugula (about 2 cups loosely packed)

sea salt

Vegetable Marinade

½ cup brown rice vinegar

2 tablespoons minced garlic

4 tablespoons olive oil

PREPARATION

Heat grill to medium-hot, or to where you can hold your hand 3 inches above the grill for 7 seconds.

Cook orzo according to package directions, drain, run under cold water, and place in large serving bowl. Add hempseed oil and stir.

Cut zucchini in half lengthwise. Cut bell pepper around core, removing seeds and white pith. Cut fennel bulb and eggplant in half lengthwise. Cut top off garlic bulb, exposing cloves, and remove outer layer of skin. Put all veggies in a baking dish or bowl along with garlic.

In a small bowl, whisk together all ingredients for vegetable marinade. Pour half the marinade onto vegetables and coat them well.

Transfer veggies to the grill. Baste veggies with remaining half of marinade while they cook. Remove veggies when done to your liking. The garlic will take the longest and can char more than the others since it's protected by skin. Once it's done, the garlic cloves will pop right out when squeezed. Let veggies cool and then roughly chop. Add to orzo in large serving bowl.

Pop garlic cloves and add them whole to the bowl. Add artichoke hearts, parsley, sesame seeds, and a pinch of salt and mix together. Add arugula and lightly mix again.

POLENTA

Polenta, or cornmeal, is the whole grain of corn that has been stone-ground. Steeped in Italian tradition, it even has its own copper preparation pot, called the paiolo. Some say polenta must be stirred constantly to reach perfection, but I have found a number of high-quality polentas that have pleased the palates of my Italian friends without requiring too much labor. Today, there are some high-quality polentas on the market that can take just 5–25 minutes to prepare, depending upon the fineness of grain, its moisture content, and the amount you are cooking.

Polenta is one of my favorite foods because of its versatility. It also brings a signature texture that adds interest to many different dishes. Always insist on organic polenta; if it is artisanally made, so much the better. Polenta, like most grains, is a real time-saver for the busy athlete; not only is it quick to prepare, but because it goes with so many foods, it is worthwhile to double the recipe and store the extra in the refrigerator for future meals.

Polenta always consists of these three basic elements, but the elements' proportions will vary depending on the particular product you are using:

polenta (stone-ground corn)
water, or chicken or vegetable stock
sea salt

Follow the instructions and, as I always suggest, prepare extra. Polenta can be used as a side dish with roasted chicken, for polenta "lasagna" or crab cakes, or with black beans (see recipes).

Polenta Crab Cakes

SERVES 2

2 cups prepared polenta

1 egg white, lightly beaten

8 ounces fresh lump crabmeat, roughly chopped

½ bunch fresh dill, chopped

1 tablespoon finely minced shallot

1 tablespoon sesame seeds, black or white

sea salt

2 tablespoons sunflower seeds (optional)

¼ cup grated raw cheese (optional)

PREPARATION

Preheat oven to 425 degrees.

Cook polenta according to instructions, but add about ⅛ cup of additional water to ensure this dish does not get too dry. Once cooked, remove from heat, add egg, and mix well. Let cool slightly and add crabmeat, dill, shallot, sesame seeds, and a pinch of salt. Mix together. Form 3–5 small patties and set on lightly oiled baking sheet.

Bake 10–15 minutes, turning halfway through.

Serve on a bed of greens with sliced tomatoes and fresh mayonnaise (see recipe on page 192) and top with cheese (optional).

VARIATION

When corn is in season, I add ½ cup fresh hulled corn kernels straight from the cob to the rest of the patty ingredients.

Polenta with Egg, Goat Cheese, and Sprouts

SERVES 1

This is a dish I can eat at any time of the day. I am lucky to be surrounded by farms where I can visit the chickens, goats, and soil that produce the ingredients. Shopping locally not only supports my local community, but the nutrient content from pasture-raised eggs and cheese is superior to that of anything produced indoors.

½ cup prepared polenta
1 large egg
2 ounces fresh raw goat cheese, crumbled
½ cup sunflower sprouts or fresh greens

PREPARATION

In a small pot, bring 2 cups water to boil. Add egg, cover, and remove from heat. Let sit in water 5 minutes for a soft yolk, 10 minutes for hard. Remove egg from water.

Crack eggshell and release egg on top of prepared polenta, followed by cheese and sprouts.

Shepherd's Polenta

SERVES 4

This is a great one-pot dish that is sure to satisfy. It is super-quick to make and great left over—just cut a slice and reheat whenever you want a quick, delicious, complete meal. It is also a dish that can follow the seasons; use whatever vegetables are available fresh.

1 cup polenta
½ cup peas, fresh or frozen
½ cup corn, fresh or frozen
1 cup sliced kale
1 tablespoon hempseed oil
1 clove garlic, minced
sea salt
½ cup grated raw cheese

PREPARATION

Preheat oven to 400 degrees.

Prepare polenta as per package instructions. If using frozen peas and corn, add them 2 minutes before polenta has finished cooking. When polenta is done, add kale, oil, garlic, and salt. If using fresh veggies, cook polenta first, remove from heat, and add vegetables, along with oil, garlic, and salt, letting everything warm through for a few minutes.

Spread polenta mixture into a glass pie pan or 9 x 9–inch baking dish. Top with cheese. Bake in oven for 15 minutes or until heated through and bubbly.

VARIATIONS

- Add leftover roasted chicken to the polenta once it has finished cooking; the residual heat will warm the chicken.
- Leftover Bolognese sauce is a great addition, or accompany with some sundried tomato spread.

Polenta "Lasagna"

SERVES 4

olive oil

3 cups prepared polenta

3 cups loosely packed fresh baby spinach, arugula, sliced kale, or chard

1½ cups raw tomato sauce or Fresh Roma Tomato Sauce (page 154)

1½ cups grated raw cheese (pecorino is delicious in this recipe)

PREPARATION

Preheat oven to 400 degrees.

Lightly oil a square 9 x 9–inch glass baking dish or bread pan. Place 1 cup cooked polenta in bottom of pan and evenly distribute. Add 1 cup greens and top with ½ cup sauce and then ½ cup cheese. Repeat layers two more times, using all the ingredients called for.

Bake 15–20 minutes, until warmed through and bubbly on top.

VARIATIONS

Use Sundried Tomato Spread (page 133), Broccoli Soup (page 110), or quick pesto instead of tomato sauce.

Raw Tomato Sauce

SERVES 4

Although it might sound like a health-driven take on an Italian classic, raw tomato sauce is a celebration of fresh produce that can be found in the annals of any Italian family's culinary heritage. Unlike a long-simmered sauce that can make use of late-season tomatoes, a raw sauce, whether blended or whole, requires peak flavor and freshness.

A basic sauce requires tomatoes, garlic, olive oil, salt, black pepper, and a choice of herbs (basil, parsley, thyme, oregano).

2 pounds fresh, ripe tomatoes (roma, beefsteak, cherry, or a mix)
3–4 tablespoons olive oil
1 clove garlic, minced
¼ cup packed herbs, torn by hand
sea salt
black pepper

PREPARATION

Make this recipe before preparing pasta or polenta, to allow the flavors to marry for as long as possible.

If necessary, remove seeds from tomatoes, then dice for larger ones or cut in half for cherry. Place in bowl with olive oil, garlic, herbs, salt, and pepper. Mix well and allow to sit. When pasta is done, drain and add to sauce, or add sauce to polenta.

VARIATIONS

- Use a mix of roma and beefsteak and place in blender with olive oil and salt. Pulse until mixture is just smooth. Too much blending will cause tomatoes to become watery.
- Add ¼ cup of sliced sundried tomatoes to diced tomatoes.
- Add ¼ cup of sundried tomatoes to food processor and blend with fresh tomatoes.

NOODLES

Who doesn't like noodles? There is something about them that makes eating fun. When made with whole grains, they are a nutritious food that you can prepare in a jiffy. Soba noodles, which hail from Japan, are traditionally made from buckwheat, a high-quality source of protein containing eight essential amino acids that the body needs to help repair tissues and build new cells. It is also an excellent source of minerals, especially magnesium, which is important for many enzymatic reactions, including ATP, the body's main energy source. In the West, buckwheat flour is typically used in pancakes, breads, and desserts.

Soba noodles are cooked the same way as pasta, generally taking 5–8 minutes to prepare. Taste as you cook, because they can become very mushy if overcooked. Add to soups, use as a base for salads, or make them an accompaniment to fish, chicken, or pork. I always make at least twice as much as I need for one meal and then use the leftovers for other things as a component for quick snacks or meals.

Cellophane noodles, also known as bean thread noodles, are a type of transparent Asian noodle made from starch. They are usually soaked in 3–4 quarts of very hot water for 10–15 minutes, then drained. Soaking time may vary depending on the thickness of the noodle and the brand you choose. Cellophane noodles readily pick up flavors from other ingredients, so they are often paired with dressings and sauces that have a little bite to them.

Soba Noodles with Baked Sesame Chicken

SERVES 2

The longer you marinate the chicken, the better the flavor—overnight is best! If time is short, cut the chicken into cubes before marinating to expedite the process.

1 pound boneless, skinless chicken breasts

2 servings prepared soba noodles

Marinade

½ cup Nama Shoyu or tamari

½ cup water

2 tablespoons fish sauce

3 tablespoons raw honey

2 tablespoons fresh lime juice

2 tablespoons fresh minced gingerroot

3 tablespoons sesame seeds

½ bunch chopped fresh cilantro leaves

PREPARATION

Whisk all marinade ingredients together in a baking dish big enough to hold and cover the chicken. Reserve ¼ cup marinade. Rinse chicken breasts in cool running water and pat dry. Place individual chicken breasts in marinade in dish. Cover the dish and refrigerate. Marinate several hours or overnight.

Preheat oven to 425 degrees.

Remove cover from baking dish and place dish on middle rack of oven. Bake 15–20 minutes or until chicken is fully cooked. If marinade cooks away, add a bit of water to the dish.

Remove dish from oven and cool slightly before cutting chicken into bite-sized pieces. Toss with reserved marinade and noodles.

Soba Noodles with Grilled Meatballs

SERVES 2

This is my Asian spin on the classic Italian dish of spaghetti and meat-balls. It has that same comfort food appeal but with a completely different flavor. Skewers of grilled meatballs are a common street food in Thailand; my addition of soba noodles provides a whole-grain source of energy and recovery nutrition for active endeavors.

2 servings soba noodles (see package for serving size)

¼ cup finely chopped scallions

1 cup fresh mung bean sprouts

Meatballs

1 pound ground beef

1 egg, lightly beaten (optional)

3 cloves garlic, minced

2 stalks lemongrass, bruised and minced

½ bunch fresh cilantro leaves, chopped

1½ tablespoons quinoa flour

2 tablespoons fish sauce

2 tablespoons toasted sesame oil

sea salt

Dressing

½ cup Nama Shoyu or tamari

2 tablespoons toasted sesame oil

2 tablespoons raw honey

2 tablespoons fresh lime juice

2 tablespoons minced fresh gingerroot

2 tablespoons sesame seeds

1 small hot pepper (bird, Thai, serrano), minced (optional)

Prepare soba noodles according to package instructions.

Preheat grill to high heat or preheat oven to 425 degrees.

Place ground beef in mixing bowl. Add egg (if using), garlic, lemongrass, cilantro, flour, fish sauce, and salt. Using your hands, mix together thoroughly. Shape into small meatballs (a bit smaller than a golf ball) and set aside on plate.

In a bowl whisk together all dressing ingredients.

For Grill

Lightly coat meatballs with sesame oil. Grill on grates approximately 7–9 minutes, for medium rare, turning often with tongs so they cook evenly. (Add more time if you like them medium well, but be careful that they don't overcook.)

For Oven

Place meatballs on a baking sheet lined with parchment paper and bake 9–11 minutes, until medium rare, or to your preference.

When meatballs are done, immediately add them to the bowl of dressing and toss well. Pour meatballs along with dressing on top of soba noodles, add scallions and bean sprouts, and toss together.

Soba Noodles with Peanut Sauce and Marinated Cucumber Salad

SERVES 2

It is hard to keep this peanut sauce in stock because it is so good. It makes preparing a tasty meal with noodles easy, and it's delicious as a dipping sauce with spring rolls, chicken wings, or meatballs. Here I have paired the noodles with a salad composed of complementary textures and flavors. Start the cucumber salad first so that the flavors can blend while you prepare the peanut sauce and noodles.

Marinated Cucumber Salad

½ cup water

2 tablespoons raw honey

3 tablespoons chopped shallot

1 tablespoon minced fresh gingerroot

1 tablespoon chopped fresh mint

½ cup brown rice vinegar

sea salt

1 large cucumber, peeled, seeded, and sliced

PREPARATION

Heat water till warm. Dissolve honey in water by whisking vigorously. While still warm, add shallots and gingerroot. Let sit until cooled. Add mint, vinegar, and a pinch of salt. Pour on top of cucumber and let marinate while preparing rest of dish.

Peanut Sauce

¼ cup raw almond butter

2 tablespoons raw peanut butter

1 tablespoon miso paste

2 tablespoons hempseed oil

2 tablespoons raw apple cider vinegar

2 tablespoons tamari

1 tablespoon fresh lime juice

1 tablespoon raw honey

1 tablespoon sesame seeds

1 tablespoon fresh gingerroot

1 small hot pepper, chopped (optional)

¼ cup fresh cilantro leaves

¼ cup chopped fresh mint leaves

¼ cup chopped fresh parsley

¼ cup water

PREPARATION

Combine all peanut sauce ingredients except water in blender or food processor and blend until smooth. Add water as necessary until sauce has a fluid consistency.

Noodles

2 servings soba noodles (see package for servings) prepared according to package instructions

½ cup finely chopped scallions

2 tablespoons black sesame seeds

½ cup dulse, torn into small pieces

½ bunch fresh parsley, chopped

PREPARATION

Put prepared noodles in a serving bowl. Add peanut sauce to noodles 1 tablespoon at a time, until noodles are well coated. Add scallions, sesame seeds, dulse, and parsley, and toss. Serve with cucumber salad.

Bean Thread Noodle Salad

SERVES 2

This dish is perfect served warm on a cool day, or served cold when it is really hot outside. I learned the basics for the dish when I was studying in Thailand, and I knew I had to create my own version as soon as I got home. Here it is.

1 package cellophane noodles (also known as mung bean noodles or bai fun)
¼ cup fresh cilantro leaves
1 tablespoon toasted sesame oil
1 tablespoon Nama Shoyu or low-sodium soy sauce
1 tablespoon fish sauce
1 tablespoon brown rice vinegar
1 teaspoon raw honey
1 tablespoon sesame seeds or hemp seeds
1 small fresh hot pepper, chopped (bird, serrano, Thai, jalapeño)
2 cups mixed fresh vegetables for steaming (I use whatever I have in the fridge), cut into bite-sized pieces

PREPARATION

Prepare noodles according to package directions. (This usually involves soaking noodles in a bowl of 3–4 quarts of very hot water for 10–15 minutes, then draining. Directions may vary from brand to brand.)

While the noodles are soaking, whisk all other ingredients except the vegetables in a small bowl and set aside while you finish preparing the rest of the salad.

Add the vegetables to the bowl of warm noodles in the last 5 minutes of soaking so they warm through. Once done, drain and return all contents to the bowl. Add dressing and toss together.

Can be served at room temperature or chilled.

- Fresh grilled shrimp, or simply add raw shrimp to noodles 5 minutes before they are done soaking and the heat of the water will cook them.
- Leftover roasted chicken or pork; this can be placed in the colander before draining the noodles to rewarm the meat.

GRAINS & LEGUMES

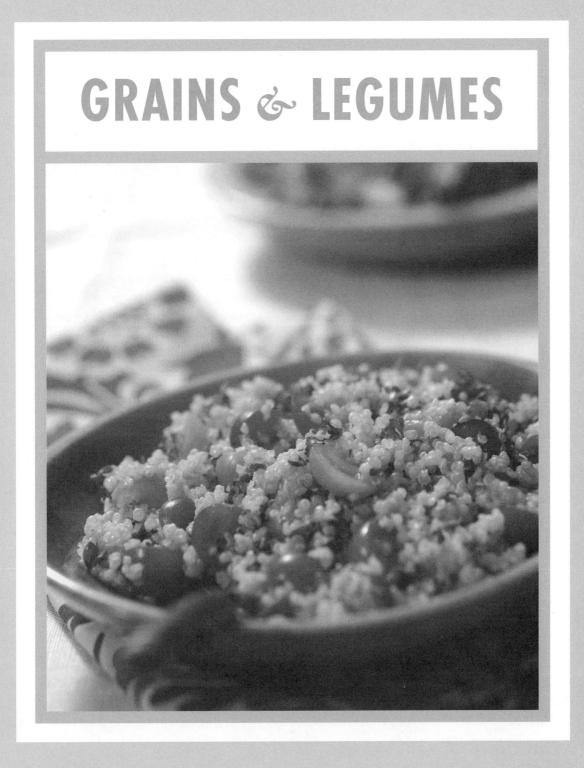

QUINOA

Originally from the Andes mountains, where it is known as the "mother of all grains," quinoa (pronounced *keen-wah*) can be found in almost every grocery store today. Quinoa is especially valuable for athletes because it is a complete protein with all of the essential amino acids that the body must obtain from food sources.

Quinoa is a great food to eat before training because of its high content of branched-chain amino acids (BCAAs), which include leucine, isoleucine, and valine, all of which are essential to aerobic metabolism. Muscles use BCAAs during exercise for the metabolism of glycogen (stored carbohydrate). As such, lower levels of BCAAs in your body can lead to less available fuel for your body during exercise.[5] In particular, leucine is effective in the secretion of insulin from the pancreas, which is responsible for the transport of blood glucose into the muscles.[6] Isoleucine helps to regulate and stabilize blood sugar and energy levels. These factors also make quinoa a good post-training meal, as it will help restore levels of BCAAs used during training. In addition, its protein-to-carbohydrate ratio of almost 4:1 will help with the repair and recovery of muscles.

Preparing quinoa is super-easy—it is made the same way you prepare rice: 2 parts water or stock (chicken or vegetable stock can be used) to 1 part grain. First rinse the raw quinoa in fresh water. Then add quinoa to a pot along with twice as much water or stock (use slightly less liquid if you are cooking at high elevation). Bring to a boil, cover, and let simmer about 15 minutes, until the water is absorbed. At that point, the grain will have uncurled and it will have a small bite similar to that of al dente pasta.

To make a smaller portion, rinse first and then combine 1 cup water with ½ cup quinoa. Bring to a boil for 5 minutes, remove from heat, and let sit, covered, for 15 minutes.

Quinoa can also be soaked for 7 to 24 hours before cooking; soaking helps break down the outer layers, making the grain more digestible and the nutrients more accessible. Add 1 tablespoon raw apple cider vinegar to 2 cups water and 1 cup quinoa. When you are ready to cook, drain and rinse, and then use the same 2:1 ratio of liquid to grain, cooking until the liquid is absorbed.

Herb Quinoa–Stuffed Tomato with Egg and Greens

SERVES 1

Quinoa may be the most versatile, healthy, and great-tasting ingredient that many people have yet to discover. Easy to prepare and easy to store, quinoa should be in everyone's pantry and diet. In this recipe, the egg's soft yolk creates a rich, silky texture and warms the dish.

1 large egg

1 cup cooked quinoa, at room temperature

1–2 tablespoons chopped fresh herbs of your choice (such as parsley, chives, mint, dill)

1 tablespoon pumpkin seed oil (hempseed or flaxseed oil works great here, too)

sea salt

1 tablespoon freshly grated raw cheese

1 medium-to-large slicing tomato (e.g., Beefsteak, Brandywine, or Cherokee), hollowed out

1½ cups greens of your choice (kale, arugula, baby spinach, or whatever you have in the kitchen)

PREPARATION

See the recipe for cooked quinoa on page 174.

Fill pot with 3–4 inches of water, enough to cover egg, and bring to a boil. Once boiling, remove from heat, place egg in water, and cover. Let sit 3–5 minutes. If using organic, free-range, or farmers' market eggs, you can let the white stay a little runny; otherwise cook the white all the way through.

While the egg cooks, toss together quinoa, herbs, oil, salt, and cheese in a small bowl. Stuff the mixture into the tomato. Place a bed of greens on a serving plate and center the stuffed tomato on top. If using a heartier green such as kale, you can use the hot water to blanch it slightly. Just make sure to clean the eggs prior to cooking, so the water is clean for blanching.

Crack the egg onto the tomato and break the yolk to let it run over the quinoa and tomato. If desired, cut up the tomato and egg mixture and toss with the greens to give everything a little more moisture before enjoying.

Quinoa Veggie Burgers

MAKES 2 BURGERS

You can bake these burgers in the oven or fry them (in just a bit of oil) on the stovetop.

1 cup flax seeds

1 cup pumpkin seeds

1 cup smoked dulse, torn into pieces

1 carrot, peeled and chopped

2 ears fresh corn, kernels sliced off

2 tablespoons chopped fresh parsley

2 tablespoons chopped shallot

1 tablespoon miso paste

2 tablespoons hempseed oil

1 tablespoon sesame seeds

sea salt

2 cups prepared quinoa (see page 174)

1 tablespoon olive oil

2 sprouted burger buns

PREPARATION

If you plan to bake the burgers, preheat oven to 400 degrees.

Soak flax seeds in 2 cups of water for 15 minutes or until all of the water has been absorbed. In bowl of food processor, place pumpkin seeds, dulse, carrot, corn kernels, parsley, shallot, miso, and hempseed oil. Pulse until mixture is ground and chunky. Add soaked flax, sesame seeds, and a pinch of salt, continuing to pulse until everything is combined. Remove from processor and place into bowl with quinoa. Mix thoroughly. Form into two patties.

To Bake

Lightly oil each side of patties with the olive oil. Place on sheet pan lined with parchment paper or place in a baking dish. Cook in oven for 10–12 minutes, turning over at the halfway point to lightly brown each side. Serve on sprouted buns.

Stovetop

Heat a skillet over medium-high heat until hot. Add 1 tablespoon of olive oil to pan and swirl to coat bottom. Place patties in pan and lightly brown on each side, about 4 minutes per side. Serve on sprouted buns.

GOOD ACCOMPANIMENTS

- Guacamole (page 138)
- Sundried Tomato Spread (page 133)
- Marinated Cucumber Salad (page 168)
- Daily Antipasto (page 120)

Quinoa Tabouleh

SERVES 4

1 cup prepared quinoa (see page 174)

1 cup halved cherry tomatoes

1½ cups packed fresh parsley leaves

1–2 tablespoons olive oil, hempseed oil, or sesame oil

juice of ½ lemon

sea salt

PREPARATION

Toss all ingredients together and serve at room temperature.

GOOD ACCOMPANIMENTS

- Grilled or roasted chicken (page 214)
- Grilled or steamed fish (page 200)
- Falafel
- Grilled vegetables
- Green salad

Toasted Kasha with Soft-Boiled Eggs and Dulse

SERVES 2

2 large eggs

½ cup toasted kasha (buckwheat groats)

½ cup smoked dulse,* torn into pieces

2 tablespoons chopped fresh parsley

pinch of red pepper flakes

sea salt

grated raw cheese

½ cup sprouts or a handful of salad greens

PREPARATION

Place eggs in a pot and cover with just enough water to submerge. Bring to a boil, remove from heat, and let stand 4 minutes.

In a separate pot, bring ½ cup water to boil, remove from heat, and add ½ cup kasha. Let stand 4–5 minutes. Cool to room temperature. Add dulse, parsley, red pepper flakes and salt; stir. Top with cheese and sprouts. Crack eggs open over top and dig in.

*Dulse is a seaweed that is full of beneficial minerals. It contains calcium, phosphorus, potassium, and sodium (which are electrolytes as well as alkalizing minerals), magnesium (good for muscles), iron (good for blood oxygen), and silica (good for joints).

Lentil Burgers

These burgers can be made fresh or using additional lentils prepared for the Black Lentil Salad (page 128).

1 cup dried black lentils or 4 cups cooked black lentils
½ cup finely chopped carrots
¾ cup raw walnuts, finely ground
1 tablespoon ground turmeric
2 teaspoons ground cumin
2 teaspoons ground coriander
2 tablespoons chopped fresh parsley
2 tablespoons chopped fresh mint leaves
2 shallots, minced
sea salt
3 tablespoons hempseed oil

PREPARATION

If preparing lentils for this recipe, rinse and sort through lentils, removing any unwanted particles. Place in medium pot, cover lentils with 2 inches of water, and bring to boil. Once boiling, turn down heat and simmer for about 30 minutes, until lentils are just past tender. Pour off any excess liquid.

Proceed from here whether using leftover or newly prepared lentils: Toss lentils with carrots and set aside to cool, if needed, on counter or in the refrigerator.

In a small bowl, toss together walnuts, turmeric, cumin, coriander, parsley, mint, shallots, and a pinch of salt. Add hempseed oil to lentils and stir. Add walnut mixture to lentils and mix together. Using your hands, form the mixture into 4 patties.

These burgers can be eaten at room temperature, or you can lightly brush them with olive oil, place on a baking sheet lined with parchment paper, and warm them in a 400-degree oven for 7–10 minutes.

GOOD ACCOMPANIMENTS

- Sprouted bread
- Tortillas
- Guacamole (pages 138–139)
- Mayonnaise (page 192)
- Sundried Tomato Spread (page 133)

Beans and Brown Rice

SERVES 4

Beans and brown rice is a dish truly fit for athletes. It is a blend of complete protein filled with plenty of fiber, vitamin B, iron, and isoflavins, all of which promote ongoing health. It makes a great pre- and post-training food, and you'd be missing a treat if you didn't have it for breakfast too, once in a while.

This recipe presents the most basic way to prepare beans. There are hundreds of varieties of beans to choose from—and they're all good—but you can use this method with any of them. I like to make a big batch of beans ahead, refrigerate, and then add various herbs and spices when I reheat them so I can change the flavors. I have been known to eat beans for three different meals in a week.

Basic Beans

1–2 cups dried beans
water to cover
2 bay leaves
2–4 garlic cloves, peeled and smashed
sea salt

PREPARATION

Sort through beans, removing any debris or small rocks. Rinse with water. Place beans in a pot and cover with water by 1–2 inches. Let soak 8 hours or overnight. (Do this in the morning before you go to work or in the evening before bed.) This will reduce the actual cooking time.

The beans will expand as they soak, so when you are ready to cook them, make sure they are covered by at least 1 inch of water. Place on stovetop, bring water to a boil, and skim foam. Allow to boil for a few minutes. Reduce heat to a gentle simmer, add bay leaves, and cover.

The beans will need to cook from 1 to 4 hours, depending on the variety. Cooking slowly over low heat, until the beans are fork-tender and produce a nice aroma, is best. In the last hour, add the garlic. Just before serving, add salt to taste. Beans can be eaten fresh along with rice or reserved along with their liquid for later use.

VARIATION

For extra flavor, dice 1 medium onion, 2 stalks of celery, and 1 large carrot (in French cooking this is called a *mirepoix*). Sauté in 1 tablespoon of olive oil with a pinch of salt for 2–3 minutes or until just soft. Add to bean pot just before cooking. To add even more flavor, add some chopped bacon or pork fat.

Basic Brown Rice

Rice comes in many different types, which are mainly distinguished by their texture and grain size (long, medium, and short). Rice is also sold according to its flavor (such as basmati and jasmine). White and brown rices are the same plant grown in paddies. All rice is composed of an outermost layer, called the husk, and an inner layer, called the bran. White rice has had both the husk and bran removed. Brown rice varieties have only had the husk removed, leaving the bran intact.

The bran is where the majority of nutrients are contained, as well as fiber, making brown rice the best choice for athletes. Brown rice's nutrients include minerals like magnesium, calcium, phosphorus, and niacin, as well as carbohydrates, fats, and protein.

Types of brown rice are determined by the amount of bran that has been retained after processing. *Fully unpolished rice* means the entire bran layer is intact, thereby giving the rice a very deep color. *Partially unpolished rice* has had a portion of the bran removed, giving it a lighter brown color.

Wild rice is not a true rice, but rather a grain harvested from grass. It grows in shallow water in lakes and streams. There are four types of wild rice: Indian (usually simply called wild rice), Texas, northern, and Manchurian. Wild rice is high in protein and low in fat and is a good source of the amino acid lysine and dietary fiber. Because of its denser grain, wild rice takes longer to cook than true rice—about 45 minutes to

1 hour—and also has a chewy texture. Presoaking will reduce the cooking time somewhat.

1 cup brown rice
2 cups water

Rinse rice 2–3 times, until water is clear. Put 2 cups of water in a medium pot; add the rice. Bring to boil, reduce heat to simmer, and cover. Simmer for 25–40 minutes, depending on the size of grain and moisture content. (Use slightly less water if you are cooking at high altitude.) When all water has evaporated, remove pot from heat, take off lid, and allow steam to escape. Transfer to bowl and fluff with fork to help separate the grains.

Note: Soaking rice (or any grain) in water, along with a bit of apple cider vinegar or whey protein, for 7–12 hours before cooking will help break down the bran and release nutrients.

SEAFOOD

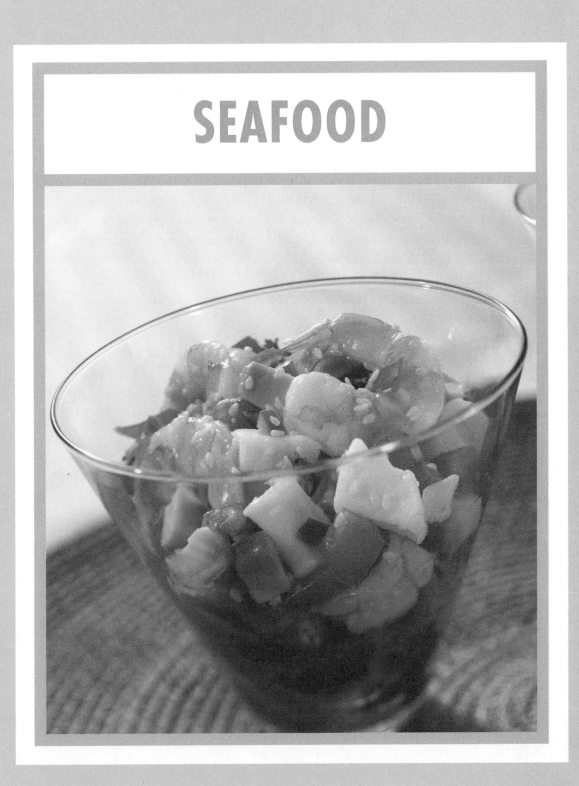

Ceviche

SERVES 2

"Ceviche! Ceviche!" I can hear my Costa Rican friend Manuel yelling out as he rides his bike up and down the beach. When it's really hot and I have just finished a long surf, paddle, or other workout, my body is not always geared up for heavy foods. But the light, refreshing, and nutritious combination of fresh fish with vegetables and a sprouted tortilla or crackers can do no wrong in my book.

1 pound firm white fish filet (such as red snapper, cod, or orange roughy), cut into chunks

1 tablespoon minced garlic

3 tablespoons diced shallot

1½ cups fresh lemon juice (the juice of about 8–10 lemons)

¾ cup fresh lime juice (the juice of about 8–10 limes)

1 jalapeño pepper, seeded and diced

½ cup diced red bell pepper

2 tablespoons chopped cilantro leaves

1 tablespoon raw sesame seeds

1 tablespoon hempseed oil

sea salt

½ cup diced tomatoes

1 avocado, diced

PREPARATION

Put fish in large stainless-steel or glass mixing bowl with garlic, shallots, and lemon juice. Refrigerate for 2½ hours. The acid in the lemon juice will slowly poach the fish. Remove, drain, and return to the bowl.

Toss with lime juice, jalapeño, red bell pepper, cilantro, sesame seeds, hempseed oil, and salt.

Spoon into 2 bowls and top with tomatoes and avocado.

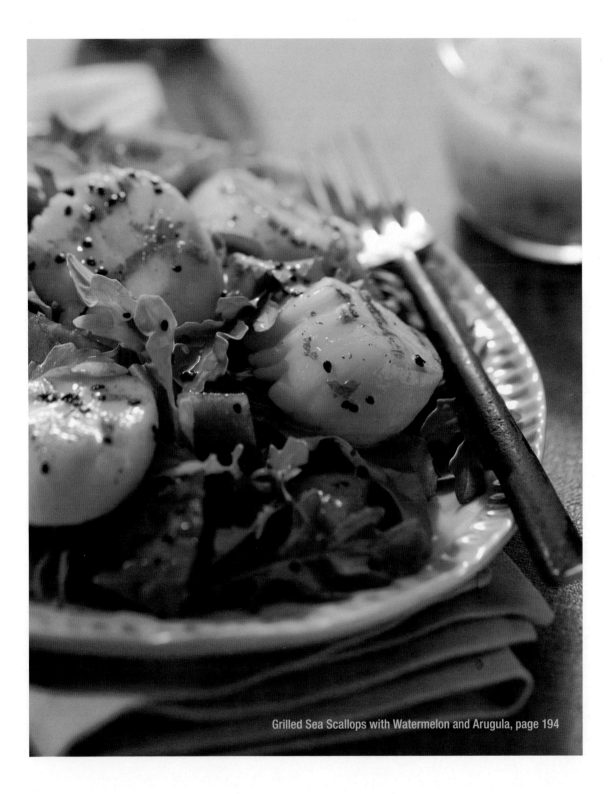

Grilled Sea Scallops with Watermelon and Arugula, page 194

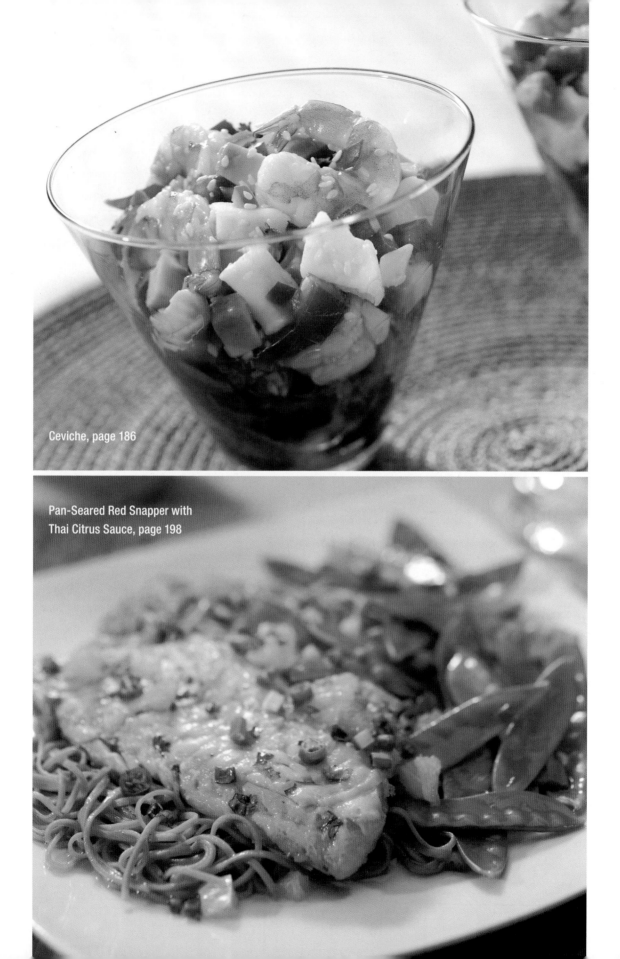

Ceviche, page 186

Pan-Seared Red Snapper with
Thai Citrus Sauce, page 198

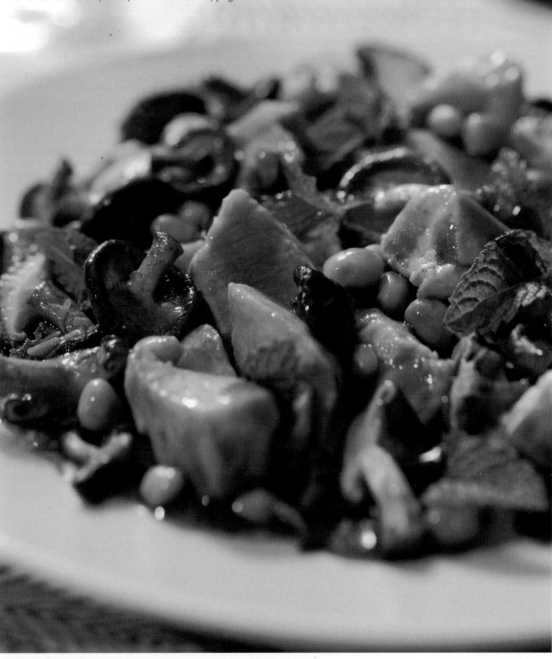
Chicken with Mint, Peas, and Mushrooms, page 208

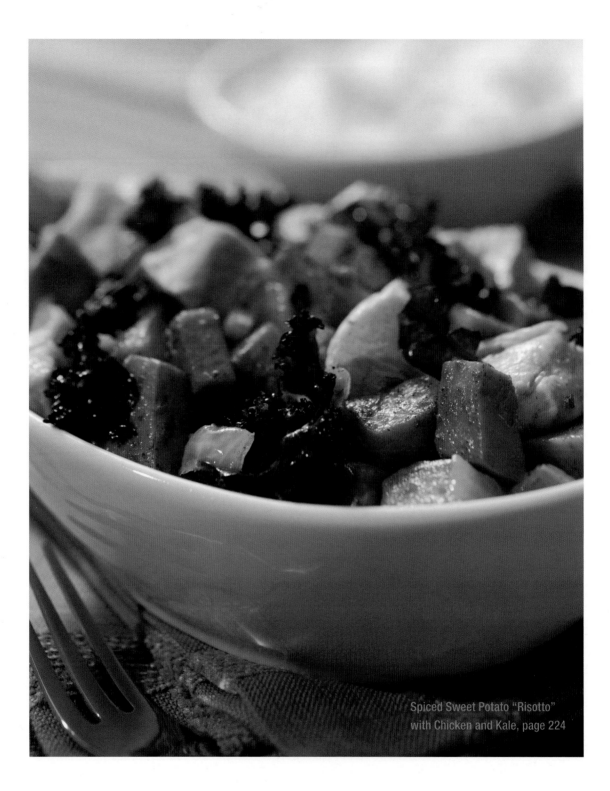

Spiced Sweet Potato "Risotto"
with Chicken and Kale, page 224

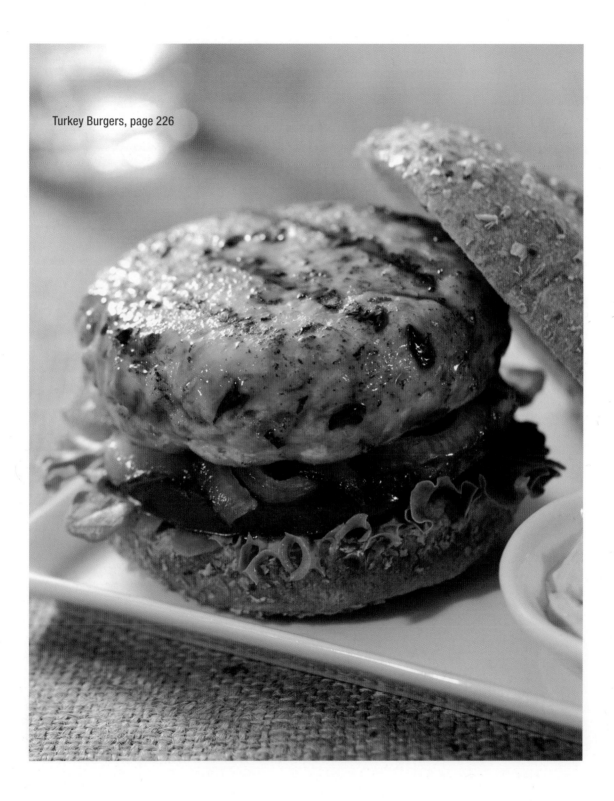

Turkey Burgers, page 226

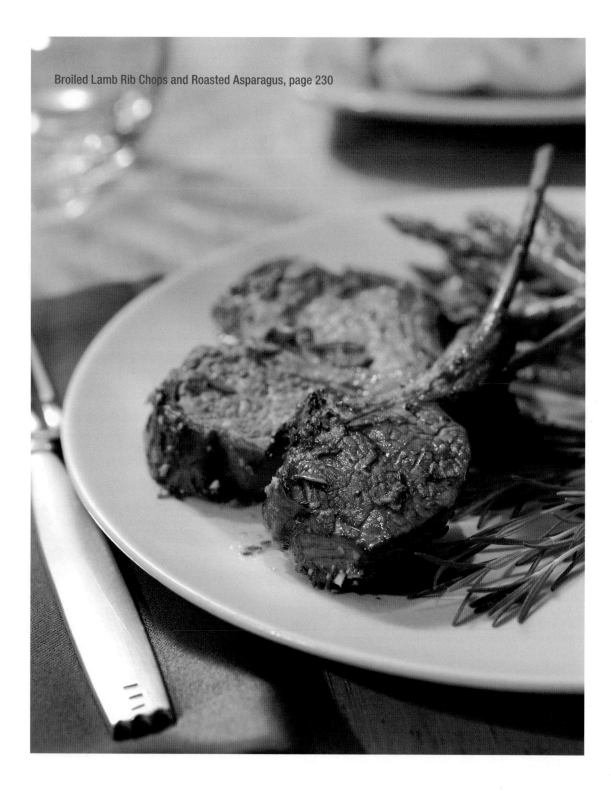
Broiled Lamb Rib Chops and Roasted Asparagus, page 230

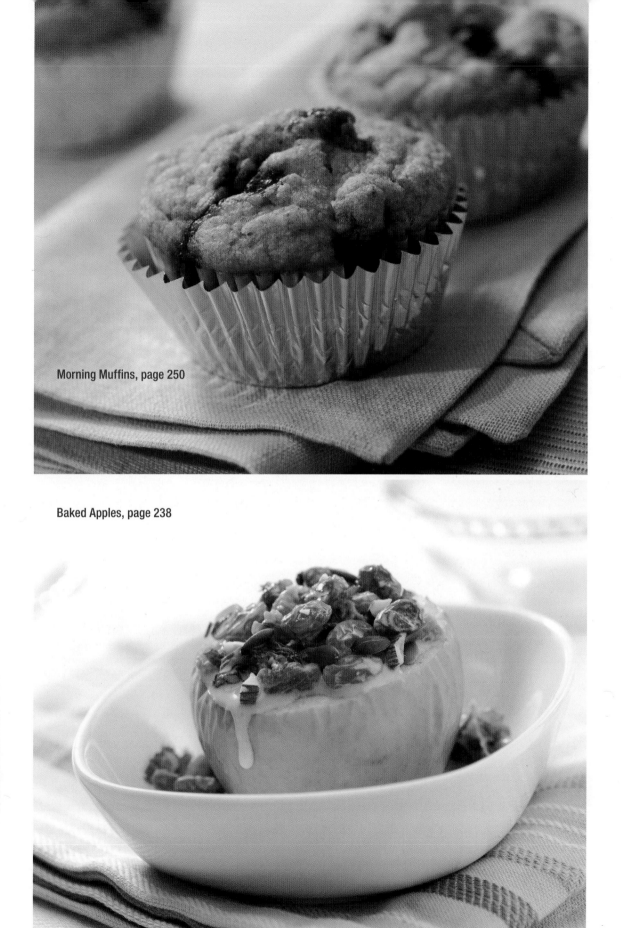

Morning Muffins, page 250

Baked Apples, page 238

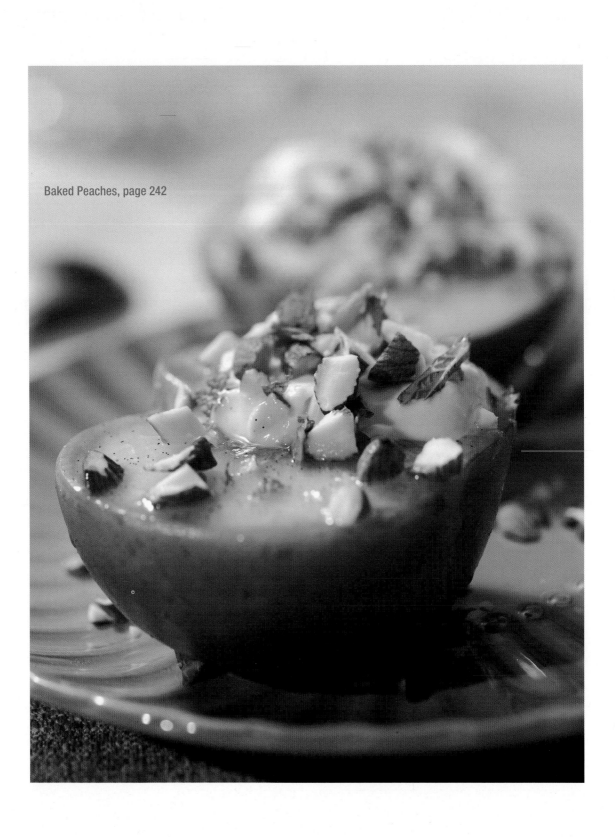

Baked Peaches, page 242

VARIATIONS

Ceviche can be made with almost any seafood, including:

- Shrimp
- Clams
- Scallops
- Lobster
- Octopus or squid
- Mussels

Fish and Vegetable Coconut Curry

SERVES 2

This is a dish I can eat at any time of the day. I normally prepare it for dinner and have leftovers for breakfast the next morning, but it is a quick and easy meal to make fresh anytime. It is a perfect combination of fats, protein, phytonutrients, and carbs. It is incredibly flavorful during the summer when corn is at its finest, but feel free to substitute frozen corn out of season.

1 tablespoon olive oil

½ medium onion, cut into chunks

1 red bell pepper, cut into chunks

1 Japanese eggplant, peeled, cut into chunks

1 tablespoon green curry paste

1 can (12–13½ ounces) whole coconut milk (make sure it has no preservatives)

1 tablespoon fish sauce

1 tablespoon raw honey

½ cup fish stock or vegetable stock

1 pound firm, whitefish fillets, skinless, at least ½ inch thick and cut into chunks (black sea bass, striper, snapper; shrimp, scallops, clams, or mussels are also good)

1 cup fresh corn kernels, cut off the cob

1 tablespoon chopped fresh cilantro

PREPARATION

Heat a large sauté pan, wok, or pot over medium-high heat. Add oil and swirl to coat bottom of pan. Add onion, bell pepper, and eggplant and sauté for 3–4 minutes. Add curry paste and sauté 2 minutes. Add coconut milk and stir to combine. Add fish sauce, honey, and stock; stir to combine. Add fish. Stir and continue cooking for 3–5 minutes, until fish is done. Add corn. Remove from heat and stir in cilantro.

Serve with cooked brown rice, quinoa, or barley groats.

Fillet of Fish en Papillote with Veggies

SERVES 2

En Papillote is a French method literally meaning "in paper," and cooking this way is simple, healthy, and flavorful. It is essentially a method of steaming inside a paper pouch that holds the ingredients. The options and flavors are endless. The only things this recipe requires are some creativity and an aversion to cleaning dishes. With those in hand, you will quickly find this to be one of your favorite cooking methods.

2 large rectangles of parchment paper (big enough to easily hold all ingredients)

2 cloves garlic, minced

2 tablespoons minced fresh gingerroot

2 tablespoons Nama Shoyu or low-sodium soy sauce

2 tablespoons toasted sesame oil

2 teaspoons raw honey

2 tablespoons sesame seeds

3 tablespoons chopped chives

1 cup green or red kale, torn into pieces

2 6- to 8-ounce fillets of fish (black sea bass, red snapper, flounder, fluke)

2 heads baby bok choy, rinsed and quartered

½ cup (4 ounces) mushrooms (shimeji, enoki, shiitake, oyster)

PREPARATION

Preheat oven to 400 degrees.

The parchment is easiest to work with if you first crumple it up into a ball and then smooth it out. Fold a sheet in half, then channel your inner second grader and cut a large heart-shaped piece from it, starting at the fold. Do the same for the other sheet. Each heart should be about 2 inches wider than the fish fillets. Set aside.

In a small bowl, whisk garlic, gingerroot, Nama Shoyu or soy sauce, sesame oil, honey, sesame seeds, and chives.

Place the parchment "hearts" open on a baking sheet. Brush half of each heart with some sesame oil and lay the kale out as the bed for the fish (the other half of the heart will be folded over and become the "lid"). Top with one fillet, then arrange bok choy and mushrooms around the fillet. Pour marinade evenly over fish and vegetables.

Fold the other half of the heart over and then crinkle and tightly roll up the exposed seam. If it refuses to stay shut, feel free to staple it closed.

Cook in oven 9–12 minutes, depending on the thickness of the fish. Thin fillets will only require 5–7 minutes. A good sign of the fish being done is the pouches puffing up with air.

Once removed from the oven, either carefully unfold the pouches or pierce with a knife to release the steam.

VARIATIONS

Although this method is most commonly used for fish, chicken works very well in its place. Cooking time will be longer.

Leftover cooked grains such as quinoa, brown rice, or buckwheat groats reheat fabulously in the steamy environment, so feel free to add a serving to each pouch as well.

Curry Version

Instead of using the mixture listed above, mix together ¼ cup coconut milk or 1 heaping tablespoon coconut butter, 1 teaspoon soy sauce, 1 teaspoon green curry paste, 1 teaspoon honey, and 1 tablespoon minced gingerroot and pour over fish. Small florets of broccoli and eggplant can be substituted for the kale, bok choy, and mushrooms.

How to make a papillote

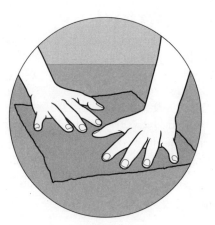

1. Crumple paper for easier handling. Smooth flat.

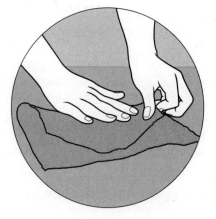

2. Fold in half horizontally.

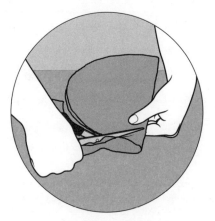

3. Cut in heart shape, leaving seam intact.

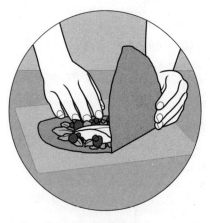

4. Place fish and vegetables on bottom half, snug against seam.

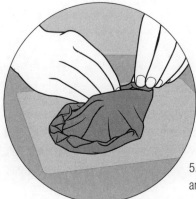

5. Roll up edges tightly, tucking in as you go, and close pouch completely.

Fresh Tuna Salad

SERVES 1

I generally avoid canned foods, and I absolutely put my foot down about canned protein, especially canned seafood. The concept of something going from the sea to a can leaves much to be desired, and the utter lack of any nutritional benefit is enough to make me pass on any convenience I might gain. My version of tuna salad is so fresh, quick, and easy, you'll never go back to the canned kind again.

Mayonnaise
2 cloves garlic
1 tablespoon lemon juice (about ½ large lemon)
2 egg yolks or 1 whole egg and 1 yolk
½ cup hempseed oil
¼ cup flaxseed oil
¼–½ cup olive oil
sea salt

Tuna
1 tablespoon olive oil
sea salt
freshly ground black pepper
8 ounces fresh tuna steak
2 tablespoons chopped fresh parsley
1 teaspoon celery seed

PREPARATION

Make the Mayonnaise
In the bowl of a food processor or a blender, combine garlic and lemon juice. Add egg yolks and briefly blend. Pour all oils into a container that has a spout (such as a liquid measuring cup), and with the motor running, slowly pour the oil into the mixture in a thin, steady stream. It's extremely important to do this slowly so the emulsion doesn't break.

Once you have incorporated all the oil, add a dash or two of salt, taste, and then season further as needed.

Note: This mayonnaise recipe makes much more than required for the tuna salad, but it's a fantastic thing to keep in an airtight container in the fridge for up to a week.

To Grill the Tuna

Preheat charcoal or propane grill to where you can hold your hand 3 inches above the grate for 3 seconds. Brush the grill grate with olive oil. Season the tuna steak(s) on both sides with a light coat of olive oil, salt, and pepper. Depending on thickness, cook each side 3–5 minutes. You do want the tuna to cook all the way through, but don't be afraid to take the tuna off the grill and let the resting heat finish the job. This will keep the tuna moist and juicy. Cool completely.

To Bake the Tuna

Preheat oven to 400 degrees. Lightly brush a glass baking dish with olive oil and cook seasoned steak(s) 10–12 minutes, turning halfway through. Cool completely.

Once tuna is cooled, place in a large mixing bowl along with any juices and break apart with two forks. Add mayonnaise a few tablespoons at a time, until the salad is moist enough for your liking. Taste for seasoning and add salt or pepper as needed. Add chopped parsley and celery seed and mix. (I'm not a fan of adding raw celery to my salad, but feel free to do so if you like the flavor.)

VARIATIONS

- Avocado-based mayonnaise: Add half an avocado in place of ¼ cup of any of the oils and increase lemon juice to 2 tablespoons. Blend egg yolks and avocado together and then add oil.
- Add some Sundried Tomato Spread (page 133) to the mix when you add the mayonnaise to the tuna.
- Make it spicy! Add some chipotle peppers or hot sauce to the mix and replace the parsley with cilantro to give the dish a southwestern flair.

GOOD ACCOMPANIMENTS

- Greens
- Mixed sprout salad with sunflower seeds
- Sprouted bread or tortillas

Grilled Sea Scallops with Watermelon and Arugula

SERVES 2

This is nothing short of a five-star gourmet meal, yet it couldn't be easier to make. From flavor to texture to appearance, this dish combines them all. The trick to its success is a clean, hot grill that has been well oiled, and a little bit of patience—once you've put the scallops on the grill, you don't want to move them too soon. This is a perfect marriage between land and sea.

1 pound medium sea scallops

1 tablespoon olive oil

sea salt

1½ cups arugula

2 cups cubed seedless watermelon (½-inch pieces)

Dressing

3 tablespoons olive oil

1 tablespoon chopped fresh mint leaves

2 tablespoons sliced scallions

1 tablespoon lime juice

1 tablespoon black sesame seeds

sea salt

1 small hot pepper (serrano, Thai, jalapeño, bird), chopped (optional)

1 tablespoon grated lime zest

PREPARATION

Rinse scallops and pat dry. Toss in a small bowl with 1 tablespoon of the olive oil and a pinch of salt. Heat a grill or grill pan until you can hold your hand 3 inches above it for 3 seconds.

While the grill heats, prepare the dressing: Whisk together 3 tablespoons olive oil, the mint, scallions, lime juice, sesame seeds, salt, and hot pepper (if using). Taste for seasoning.

Brush the grill with some olive oil and cook scallops about 4 minutes on each side, until they turn white the entire way through and are slightly springy to the touch. Set aside to cool while you finish the salad.

In the same bowl used for the dressing, toss the arugula and watermelon in the dressing, and then add the scallops. Transfer to a plate and garnish with lime zest.

Island Grilled Shrimp

SERVES 2

Shrimp sizes are determined by how many are in a pound. For example, "25/30" means there are between 25 and 30 shrimp in each pound. I find those in the "15/20" range best. They have a nice sweetness and texture and are easy to manage with their shells on. The shrimp business has become a big global industry, and shrimp are often sprayed with a chemical preservative to help maintain their integrity over long-distance travel. For this reason I only buy them when they are fresh and domestic.

1 pound shrimp, peeled, deveined, rinsed, and patted dry

Island Rub
1 tablespoon olive oil

1 tablespoon stone-ground or coarse-ground mustard

1 tablespoon raw honey

1 tablespoon ground turmeric

sea salt

2 teaspoons red pepper flakes

2 tablespoons whole coriander seeds

2 tablespoons whole cumin seeds

1 tablespoon minced fresh gingerroot

1 tablespoon minced garlic

2 tablespoons chopped fresh parsley

juice of ½ lemon

Special Tools
Spice grinder or mortar and pestle

PREPARATION
Heat grill until you can hold your hand 3 inches above the grate for 3 seconds, or preheat oven to 425 degrees.

While the grill or oven heats, place prepared shrimp in a medium-sized mixing bowl. Set aside.

In a small bowl, whisk olive oil, mustard, and honey together. Add turmeric, a pinch of salt, and crushed red pepper flakes. Whisk to combine. Using a spice or coffee grinder or mortar and pestle, grind coriander and cumin seeds to powder and add to mixture. Pour mixture over shrimp and toss well. Add the ginger and garlic, and toss again.

To Grill

Lightly brush grill with oil. Place shrimp on grates, working quickly. Cook on grill for 2–3 minutes on each side or until pink and no longer translucent. Toss the cooked shrimp with parsley and lemon juice and serve immediately.

To Bake

Place shrimp on large baking sheet lined with parchment paper. Place on center rack of oven and cook 5–9 minutes, flipping halfway through. Shrimp will be pink and opaque when done.

VARIATIONS

The island rub for this recipe can just as easily be used on fish (from flounder to tuna) as well as for grilled, baked, or roasted chicken or pork.

Note: If you use your coffee grinder to grind the spices, be sure to clean it before and after by emptying the bowl and then grinding some torn-up pieces of fresh bread in the grinder. This not only cleans the grinder but also absorbs all the oils from the coffee and spices to prevent cross-saturation of flavors.

Pan-Seared Red Snapper
with Thai Citrus Sauce

SERVES 2

2 6- to 8-ounce fillets red snapper (or other firm whitefish, such as black sea bass)
sea salt
1 tablespoon olive oil

Thai Citrus Sauce

1 whole lime, sectioned, juices reserved
1 whole orange, sectioned, juices reserved
1 whole lemon, sectioned, juices reserved
¼ cup Nama Shoyu or low-sodium soy sauce
¼ cup brown rice vinegar
¼ cup raw honey
¼ cup water
2 tablespoons chopped cilantro
1–3 Thai chili peppers
2 tablespoons thinly sliced scallions

PREPARATION

Preheat oven to 425 degrees.

Make the citrus sauce first. Roughly chop the sections of lime, orange, and lemon and place in a bowl, reserving as much juice as possible. In a small bowl, whisk together Nama Shoyu or soy sauce, vinegar, honey, and water. Add the chopped citrus and juices along with cilantro, peppers, and scallions, and stir.

Heat an ovenproof sauté pan over medium-high heat on the stove. Sprinkle salt on both sides of fish. When the pan is hot, add olive oil and swirl around bottom of pan. Place fillets, skinside down, in pan and gently shake to prevent from sticking. Cook untouched for 5–7 minutes while the skin crisps. When the fillets can be easily turned over, flip them with a spatula and cook 1–2 minutes. Remove pan from heat and place in oven for 5 minutes to finish. Transfer fillets to a platter or 2 plates.

- Soba noodles
- Steamed kale
- Steamed snow peas

How to segment an orange

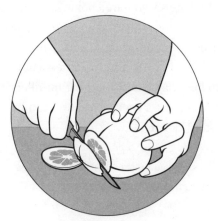

1. Using a thin paring knife, slice off orange ends.

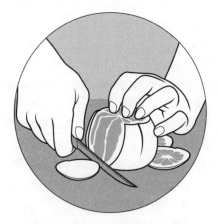

2. Place orange cut side down to steady. Cut off skin by running knife around edge. Avoid cutting flesh.

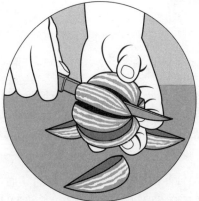

3. Carefully slice along membrane walls toward center of fruit to release each segment, leaving membrane behind.

Steamed Fish with Garlic, Ginger, and Lime

SERVES 2

Steaming is one of my favorite culinary techniques because it is easy to do and it accentuates the fresh flavors of whatever you are cooking. Fish is a perfect food to steam because steaming helps retain its moisture. I also use the water to prepare noodles, adding aromatics that flavor the fish as well as make a base for broth (see "Variations"). Bamboo steamers come in a variety of sizes, from miniature to fairly large and are great for fillets or a whole fish. They are reasonably priced, last a good while, and can be composted when they do eventually break down.

1 whole fish, 2–2½ pounds, cleaned with scales removed (red snapper, black sea bass, striper, or any local whitefish)
2 cloves garlic, minced
1 tablespoon minced fresh gingerroot
2–3 large pieces kombu kelp seaweed or banana leaf
1 lime, half sliced thin, the other half reserved
¼ cup cilantro leaves
sea salt

PREPARATION

Rinse fish and pat dry. Make 3 diagonal slices into each side of fish about 1½ inches in length and almost to the bone. Mix garlic and ginger together with a pinch of salt and evenly rub into fish slits. Line steamer basket with kombu or banana leaf. Place fish on this layer and top with slices of lime.

In a pot that is wide enough to hold the steamer, bring 3 inches of water to a boil. Reduce heat to simmer, place steamer in pot, cover, and steam fish for 10–15 minutes, depending on thickness. After 10 minutes you can uncover the steamer and check for doneness by pulling at the slits lightly and looking toward the bone. When finished, the fish will no longer look translucent and will easily flake off the bone.

Remove steamer from pot and place on top of cutting board. You can easily lift the fish out of the steamer using the kombu or banana leaf and then slide it onto a platter. Remove the lime slices and squeeze the juice of the remaining half of lime over fish. Garnish with cilantro leaves.

VARIATIONS

Add aromatics to the water: whole cloves of garlic, sliced gingerroot, a few pieces of star anise, bruised lemongrass, parsley or cilantro stalks, or some slices of lime or lemon. Be creative; the additions will add flavor to your fish.

Wrap the whole fish in banana leaves and grill for 7 to 10 minutes on each side.

GOOD ACCOMPANIMENTS

I like to use the steaming water to reheat leftover soba noodles. Dress them with a splash of Nama Shoyu, some sesame seed oil, and a pinch of red pepper. Or pour the water over sliced kale greens, lightly blanching them. Accompany with cooked grain, such as couscous, quinoa, or rice.

Tuna Tartare

SERVES 2

In the summer, when tuna is in season, it comes into my local seafood shop as fresh as can be. Less than two days out of the water makes for a melt-in-your-mouth experience. I often eat it with a dab of Nama Shoyu or olive oil and salt, but when I have guests this is the recipe I use.

1 pound fresh tuna
1 tablespoon olive oil
1 tablespoon minced fresh tarragon
1 tablespoon minced fresh chives
1 tablespoon minced fresh gingerroot
1 tablespoon minced shallot
1 tablespoon sesame seeds
1 tablespoon hempseed oil
sea salt
juice of ½ lemon
2 tablespoons lemon zest
1 tablespoon chopped fresh parsley
fresh greens, The Essential Salad (page 126), or cooked grain

PREPARATION

Chop or dice tuna into small pieces: cut the steak into ⅛-inch-thick pieces, stack a few of them, and cut ⅛-inch strips (julienne), then dice into cubes. Add to a mixing bowl. Starting with the olive oil, add the rest of the ingredients through the hempseed oil one at a time, turning the tuna after each addition to coat it well. Once the herbs have been incorporated, add a pinch of salt. Do not add the lemon juice, zest, or parsley yet.

Prepare plates with a bed of fresh greens, Essential Salad, or grain. Just before serving, mix in lemon juice. Sprinkle with lemon zest and parsley.

GOOD ACCOMPANIMENTS

- The tuna tartare is delicious as a topping on whole-grain chips.
- For an Asian-style taco, fill half-sheets of dried sushi nori with tartare.

Whole Baked Fish

SERVES 2–3

Cooking whole fish is different from cooking fillets because the bones help retain moisture and flavor. Leftovers from this recipe are great in spring rolls, sandwiches, and soups, or on top of salad greens. The bones as well as the head can be used to make fish stock.

3–5 garlic cloves, crushed
1 whole 2–3 pound fish (striped bass, black sea bass, or anything local to your waters), cleaned with scales removed
4 tablespoons olive oil, divided
sea salt
2 Japanese eggplants, cut lengthwise and then into wedges
1 cup freshly shelled peas

PREPARATION

Preheat oven to 400 degrees.

Take one clove of smashed garlic and rub it all over the fish on both sides. Make 3 diagonal cuts about ½ inch apart and almost to the bone on each side of the fish. Place bits of smashed garlic inside cuts as well as in belly. Rub fish all over with 1 tablespoon of olive oil. Sprinkle salt on both sides.

Mix 2 tablespoons of olive oil with eggplant and a pinch of salt. In a separate bowl, mix remaining 1 tablespoon of oil with peas and a pinch of salt.

Place prepared fish in baking dish and set in oven on middle rack. Total cooking time will be between 15 and 25 minutes, depending upon thickness of fish. After 7–10 minutes, add eggplant to dish, surrounding the fish. After another 5–10 minutes, add peas (these need only 3–5 minutes' cooking time or they will become mushy). When fish is done, the juices will run clear, and the meat will be opaque and will flake off the bone.

Remove fish from the baking dish using a spatula and place on platter. Add ¼ cup water to baking dish and scrape any fish drippings from the bottom of the pan with a wooden spoon. Arrange vegetables around fish and pour drippings over.

Serve with cooked grain and fresh greens or Daily Antipasto (page 120).

Steamer Bowls

SERVES 1

These bowls are two of my favorite dishes. I created them to simplify my cooking as well as to reduce the number of dishes I need to clean. They are super-easy to prepare, require very little equipment, take almost no time to cook, are always beautiful and healthy, and have tons of creative variations that make them decidedly different.

Steamer bowls are the antithesis of any kitchen work that involves sautéing. Both dishes below are made up of simple components. It's how you put them together that allows for creativity and personal flair.

Equipment

1 ovenproof bowl per person

A 3-quart or larger saucepan, casserole, stockpot, or sauteuse

ASIAN VERSION

6 ounces firm fish, cubed into ½-inch pieces (e.g., monkfish, halibut, snapper, or sea bass)

½ cup cooked quinoa, brown rice, soba noodles, mung bean pasta, or rice noodles

2 cups kale (red Russian, green, lacinato, or mix), tatsoi, bok choy, green chard, or any other leafy green of your liking

Marinade/Dressing

½ tablespoon toasted sesame oil

2 tablespoons tamari

½ tablespoon minced garlic

½ tablespoon minced fresh gingerroot

1 tablespoon chopped cilantro leaves

½ teaspoon raw honey or agave nectar

1 teaspoon sesame seeds

1 teaspoon red pepper flakes (optional)

PREPARATION

Whisk all marinade ingredients together in a bowl; add the fish.

Place ½ cup of leafy greens in bottom of an ovenproof bowl. Top with grain or noodles. Arrange remainder of greens around outside of bowl and grains. Alternate with red and green kale, or tuck stem side of tatsoi or bok choy into grain.

Spread fish on top of grain. Pour remaining marinade over fish and greens.

Add ½ inch water to the pot. Bring to rolling simmer. Place bowl in center of pot and cover. (If preparing several bowls at once, arrange bowls in pot as needed.) Steam 7–10 minutes. Remove bowl from pot with tongs and serve.

ITALIAN VERSION

6 ounces fresh fish, as above
½ cup precooked pasta that is slightly underdone, or use fresh pasta
1½ cups packed broccoli rabe, kale, or other hearty leafy green

Marinade/Dressing

½ tablespoon olive oil
2 tablespoons fresh lemon juice
½ tablespoon minced garlic
1 tablespoon chopped fresh parsley
sea salt

PREPARATION

Follow instructions for the Asian version.

POULTRY

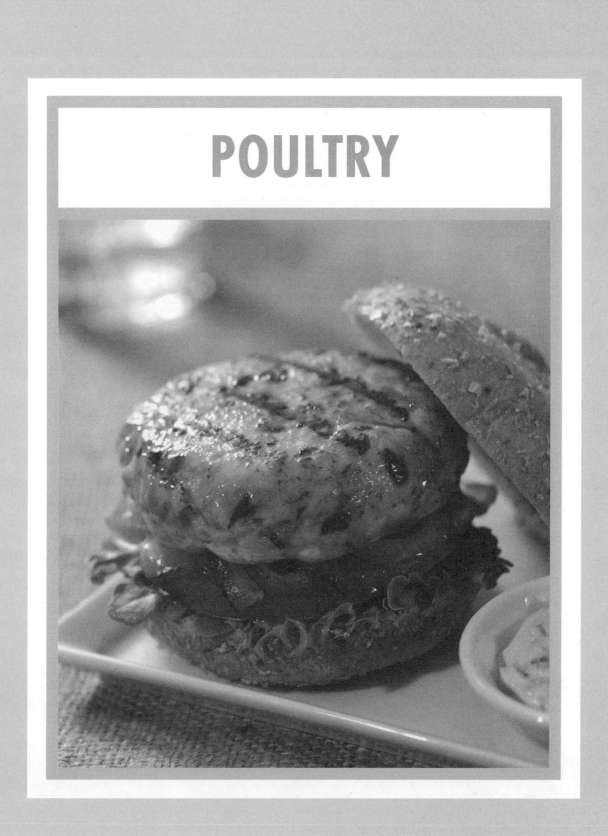

Chicken with Mint, Peas, and Mushrooms

SERVES 2

This is a wonderful spring dish when the peas are sweet and the mushrooms fresh. Once peas are picked, their sugars begin to turn to starch and they begin to lose their flavor, so be sure to use them right away. Fresh raw peas are delicious, so make sure you have bought enough to eat some as you shell them, or else there won't be enough to make it to the pan!

2 tablespoons olive oil

1 tablespoon unsalted butter

1 pound boneless chicken breasts, cubed

sea salt

2 cloves garlic, minced

1 cup freshly shelled peas

1 cup fresh morels, shiitakes, or blue oyster mushrooms, cleaned and trimmed

¼ cup water

1 teaspoon arrowroot powder (optional)

3 tablespoons chopped fresh mint leaves

PREPARATION

Heat sauté pan over medium-high heat. Add olive oil and butter. Once butter foaming has subsided, add chicken and sprinkle with salt. Sauté chicken until almost cooked through, about 3–4 minutes, constantly stirring to prevent the chicken from clumping together.

Add the garlic and continue to stir 2 minutes. Add the peas and mushrooms and cook 1–2 minutes. Add the water. Using a wooden spoon, scrape up all the browned bits on the bottom of the pan.

Bring the liquid in the pan to a boil and add the arrowroot powder if you'd like a thicker sauce. Stir well and the sauce will immediately thicken. The longer you cook it, the thicker the sauce will become, so check the chicken for doneness and gauge how thick you'd like your sauce to be from there.

Remove from heat, stir in the mint, and divide onto 2 plates.

GOOD ACCOMPANIMENTS

- Brown rice (page 183)
- Quinoa (page 174)

Chicken Satay

SERVES 2

You can prepare these skewers in the oven or on the grill. I like to serve them with fresh, crisp leaves of lettuce that I use to pull the meat off, but of course they are great on their own.

1 pound boneless, skinless chicken breasts
½ cup coconut milk
1 teaspoon fish sauce
1 teaspoon honey
1 teaspoon ground cumin
1 teaspoon ground coriander
1 teaspoon ground turmeric
1 tablespoon minced fresh gingerroot
sea salt
bamboo skewers
lettuce leaves for serving (optional)

Dipping Sauce
½ cup coconut milk
2 tablespoons red curry paste
2 tablespoons miso paste
½ cup chunky raw peanut butter or almond butter
½ cup chicken stock
2 tablespoons raw honey
2 tablespoons fresh lime juice
1 tablespoon fish sauce
1 tablespoon minced fresh gingerroot
1 tablespoon chopped cilantro
sea salt

PREPARATION

Submerge bamboo skewers in water for 2 hours or longer.

Cut chicken into ½-inch chunks. Mix together coconut milk, fish sauce, honey, ginger root, and spices. Marinate the chicken in this for 2 hours or overnight. (If you want to bake the chicken, then marinate either whole breasts or chunks in a baking dish.)

Combine all ingredients for dipping sauce in a medium pan; place over stove on medium heat. Stir while heating for 5 minutes. Remove from heat.

If grilling, start grill. If baking, preheat oven to 400 degrees.

Thread marinated chicken onto skewers, 5–7 pieces each. Place skewers on grill and cook 3–4 minutes on each side. If baking, place chicken in baking dish on middle rack and cook 12–15 minutes. Remove from grill or oven and serve with dipping sauce.

GOOD ACCOMPANIMENTS

- Marinated Cucumber Salad (page 168)
- The Essential Salad (page 126)
- Peanut sauce from soba noodles (page 169)

Grilled or Baked Chicken Wings with Garlic and Parsley

SERVES 4

Sharing a big pile of chicken wings with friends after a long day of play or training can be glorious. Gathering around the grill enhances the experience, but these wings can also be baked in the oven. The wings are not the leanest part of the chicken, but cooking them over a low flame on the grill renders some of the fat, and the skin is not only tasty but quite good for you.

2 pounds chicken wings

½ cup olive oil

2 tablespoons brown rice vinegar

5–6 garlic cloves, minced

¼ cup chopped fresh parsley

½–1 tablespoon red pepper flakes (optional)

sea salt

½ tablespoon fresh lime juice (about ½ lime)

PREPARATION

Cut wings into 3 pieces at the joints (I give my dogs all of the wing tips) and place in mixing bowl. In a separate bowl, whisk together oil, vinegar, garlic, parsley, red pepper, and salt. Taste for seasoning. Set aside ¼ cup of mixture and pour the rest over the chicken. Toss and massage into chicken with hands. Cover and let marinate in fridge 45 minutes or overnight.

To Grill

Heat grill until your hand can be 3 inches above the grate for 7 seconds. Brush grill with olive oil. Place wings on grill skinside down and cook slowly for about 10 minutes on each side, until done.

To Bake

Preheat oven to 375 degrees. Line a baking sheet with foil and arrange marinated wings on it. Bake for 30–45 minutes or until done, tossing halfway through.

Toss hot wings with reserved dressing and lime juice in large mixing bowl. Serve.

VARIATION: ASIAN-STYLE SAUCE

½ cup Nama Shoyu or low-sodium soy sauce

¼ cup water

3 tablespoons fish sauce

2 tablespoons toasted sesame oil

2 tablespoons brown rice vinegar

1 tablespoon fresh lime juice

1 tablespoon raw honey

3 cloves garlic, smashed

1 inch fresh gingerroot, peeled and thinly sliced

2 tablespoons chopped fresh cilantro

PREPARATION

Whisk all ingredients in large mixing bowl. Salt should be unnecessary due to the fish sauce and Nama Shoyu, but adjust seasonings to taste. Reserve ¼ cup of dressing and toss the wings with the rest. Marinate 45 minutes to overnight, then grill as instructed above. Toss hot wings with reserved dressing.

Oven-Roasted Chicken with Four Aromatic Variations

SERVES 4

Whole roasted chicken is one of the great American classics, and it will make any home cook feel like an almighty chef. The task might seem daunting, but for someone with an active lifestyle a roasted chicken can be the cornerstone for multiple meals. For a family it can feed everyone, and for entertaining it is a surefire winner. Although there are hundreds of recipes and techniques, this one is simple, great-tasting, and comes out perfect every time.

For active athletes, one of the best things about this recipe is that after the chicken is in the oven, there's no need to touch it or think about it until it is done. While it is cooking you can prepare some side dishes, such as polenta or salad, help the kids with homework, or even get in a quick workout. You can also base a number of meals around it for your week ahead.

If you have a metal cooking rack for your roasting pan, you can use it to support the bird. I prefer to make a rack from vegetables, which I simply cut up and distribute in the pan before placing the bird on top, and this is the method I recommend.

1 3- to 3½-pound organic, free-range roasting chicken
sea salt
freshly ground black pepper (optional)
1 tablespoon olive oil

For the Cooking Rack the Bird Will Sit On
2 carrots, peeled and cut in half
2 stalks celery, trimmed
1 medium onion, peeled and quartered

Special Tools

Kitchen twine

AROMATIC VARIATIONS

Perfect for Autumn

½ Anjou pear, halved

½ lemon, quartered

1 bunch fresh rosemary (about 4–5 sprigs)

3–4 whole garlic cloves, slightly crushed

sea salt

freshly ground black pepper

Simple and Tangy

½ lemon, quartered

1 bunch fresh parsley (about 4–5 sprigs)

½ garlic bulb

sea salt

freshly ground black pepper

Asian-Inspired

2 stalks lemongrass, bruised and trimmed

2–3 1-inch pieces fresh gingerroot, peeled

1 bunch cilantro

1 lime, cut in half

1 tablespoon toasted sesame oil

2 tablespoons tamari or soy sauce

Smoky and Spicy

1 tablespoon ground cumin

1 tablespoon ground coriander

½ tablespoon ground turmeric

1 tablespoon paprika

3–4 garlic cloves

sea salt

freshly ground black pepper

PREPARATION

Preheat oven to 400 degrees with oven rack in middle.

Cut 2 pieces of kitchen twine of about an arm's length (you can always cut off excess) for trussing.

Rinse chicken with cold water and then pat dry inside and out. Liberally sprinkle salt and pepper inside the cavity and then stuff in whichever aromatics you've selected. I like to put the garlic in first so it really permeates the chicken. Feel free to leave the giblets and neck in as well (wash and dry first); they will add flavor.

Rub the skin of the chicken with the olive oil. (You needn't feel compelled to oil the skin; there should be enough fat in the skin to do the job, but the oil will add flavor and crispness.) Liberally sprinkle salt (and pepper, if you like) over the exterior of the bird, making sure to get some between the legs and breast as well as the crevices around the wings.

To truss the chicken, which will help it cook evenly, tuck the tips of the wings close to the body. With the chicken breast side up, slide 1 piece of kitchen twine underneath (across the back) at the midpoint of the wings and then tie snugly on top. Slide the other piece of twine underneath and at the midpoint of the thighs. Bring the legs up and cross them over, covering the cavity opening as well as possible. Bring the ends of the twine from under the crossed legs and tie in a tight bow. Don't worry about tying it too tightly; the chicken will shrink when it cooks, and cutting the string will be easy.

Arrange the rack vegetables on the bottom of a roasting pan and lay the bird gently on top.

Place pan in center of preheated oven and set the timer for 1 hour and 15 minutes. When the time is up, remove the chicken from the oven. You can use a meat thermometer to check the temperature of the leg, which should be 160

How to truss a whole chicken

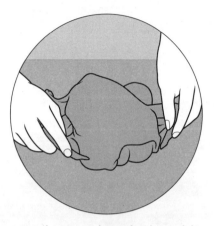

1. Bend wings under and tuck in tightly.

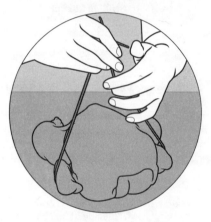

2. Slide kitchen string under front of bird and bring it up tightly.

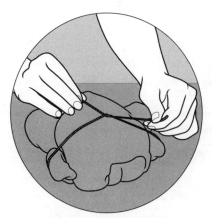

3. Tie a knot across breast.

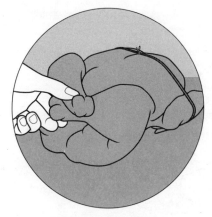

4. Cross legs in front of cavity.

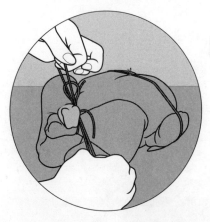

5. Loop string under legs and tie them tightly together.

degrees when done. Alternatively, you can cut into the bird at the leg joint. If the juices run clear, you're good to go.

Once the chicken is done, set it on a cutting board. Let rest at least 10 minutes and then remove twine with scissors or a knife. Using a sharp chef's knife, cut along the leg joints by pulling back the leg where the thigh meets the breast, and remove the leg (you can also probably pull the leg away with your hands, but this will tear the skin; using a knife ensures a clean cut). Repeat on other side. Remove the wings in the same way, pulling them away from the body and cutting through the joint. You can use kitchen shears instead of a knife if you prefer.

For the breast, slide a knife along the bird's spine, and you'll easily feel where the breast separates. Slowly cut down into the breast along the spine, letting the bones guide you where to cut. Use your fingers to pry the meat away from the bones (careful, it's hot!) and then continue with your knife to carve the meat.

Alternatively, you can use kitchen shears to remove the breast, keeping the meat on the bone. Start from the cavity opening and cut through the center of the breast. Then cut down along the contour of the breast where it meets the ribs, and then back up to the neck. Repeat on other side.

You can prepare a sauce while the chicken rests or let a spare set of hands prepare it while you carve the chicken. To make it, spoon off the excess fat from the pan and place pan over medium-high heat on the stove. Add ½ cup water or chicken stock, stirring and scraping up all the delicious bits on the bottom with a wooden spoon while bringing to a boil. Reduce heat and simmer 5 minutes or so, until liquid is slightly reduced. Taste for seasoning. You can serve the rack vegetables with the sauce, remove them, or crush and blend them to create thicker sauce.

How to carve a chicken

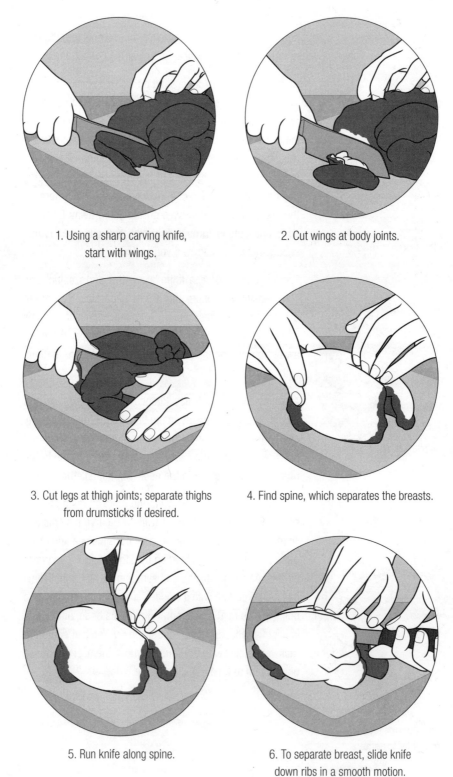

1. Using a sharp carving knife, start with wings.

2. Cut wings at body joints.

3. Cut legs at thigh joints; separate thighs from drumsticks if desired.

4. Find spine, which separates the breasts.

5. Run knife along spine.

6. To separate breast, slide knife down ribs in a smooth motion.

- Roasted root vegetables: Right after the bird goes in the oven, chop up some root vegetables—beets, carrots, turnips, potatoes, onions—into 1- to 2-inch chunks, or quartered. Toss with extra-virgin olive oil, salt, and black pepper. Add some dried or fresh herbs (rosemary, thyme, savory). Add to roasting pan 15 minutes into cooking.
- Polenta

VARIATIONS

- Use the meat in spring rolls (page 222), sandwiches, or soba noodle soup.
- Use the leftover chicken carcass to make stock: Fill a 4-quart pot with filtered water. Add the leftover chicken carcass along with aromatics and any leftover veggie ends from the main recipe. Add 1–2 tablespoons apple cider vinegar to help extract calcium and collagen from the bones. Bring the water to a simmer and leave on the stove 1–3 hours, or up to 12 hours, adding water as needed so the chicken is always covered. Strain the stock and immediately cool as rapidly as possible. Store in airtight containers in the fridge up to 2 weeks, or freeze in ice cube trays, then store in plastic freezer bags up to 2 months. This stock has many uses, such as cooking grains or making polenta, can be used for soups such as miso, or can be heated and enjoyed by itself.

Chicken with Green Beans, Tomatoes, and Pasta

SERVES 2

4 ounces pasta of your choice

2 tablespoons olive oil

1 tablespoon butter

1 pound boneless, skinless chicken breast, cubed

sea salt

2 tablespoons minced garlic

1½-ounce jar anchovies, chopped (optional)

½ pint cherry tomatoes, halved

red pepper flakes (optional)

½ pound green beans, rinsed and trimmed

2 tablespoons chopped fresh parsley

½ cup grated raw cheese

PREPARATION

Bring a large pot of salted water to a boil and cook pasta according to directions.

While the pasta cooks, heat a sauté pan over medium-high heat. Add olive oil and butter to pan, and heat until the foam from the butter subsides. Add chicken and sprinkle liberally with salt. Cook chicken almost completely through, about 3–5 minutes, stirring occasionally. Add the garlic and cook 1 minute, until fragrant. Reduce heat. Add the anchovies, if using, and cook 30 seconds, then add tomatoes and red pepper flakes if desired.

When the pasta is about 2 minutes away from being done, toss the green beans into the water. Let them cook along with the pasta while it finishes, then drain the pot. Pour pasta and beans into the pan with the chicken and toss to combine.

Garnish each serving with parsley and grated cheese.

Pan-Roasted Chicken

SERVES 4

1 whole chicken, cut into 8 pieces (you can ask your butcher to do this for you)
sea salt
1 tablespoon olive oil

PREPARATION

Preheat oven to 425 degrees.

Liberally salt skin side of chicken. Heat oil in large pan for 2–3 minutes over medium-high heat. (Use a pan that is ovenproof and large enough to hold all of the chicken so that the pieces are not touching each other.)

Once oil is hot, place chicken in pan skinside down. Put the breast in first, followed by the legs, thighs, and then the wings. This gives the thicker pieces some time to begin cooking. Shake the pan back and forth while doing so in order to prevent the chicken from sticking.

Cook chicken untouched in pan for 7–9 minutes. Avoid lifting to peek at doneness, or the skin will detach from the meat. Once ready, the pieces will easily turn over, revealing a golden brown color.

Cook on second side for 1–3 minutes and then place pan in oven. Roast 15–20 minutes. Remove from oven and place chicken pieces on platter to rest.

While the chicken rests, spoon off extra fat and heat pan over medium-high heat. Add ¼ cup water and bring to a boil while scraping brown bits off pan with wooden spoon. When bottom of pan is clean and water has slightly reduced, pour it on top of chicken.

GOOD ACCOMPANIMENTS

- Whole grains
- Greens
- Blanched broccoli or cauliflower

Spring Rolls with Vegetables and Chicken

SERVES 2 (MAKES 4 ROLLS)

The first time I saw vendors preparing spring rolls in the streets of Bangkok, I stood amazed at how simple they were to prepare. When I took my first bite, I was hooked forever. The combination of texture and freshness of flavors wrapped in a delicate piece of rice paper immediately won me over. These are great for a small meal during the day or to have as something light and fresh before or after a workout, when you don't feel like eating anything heavy. As an option, I suggest using a "spiralizer" to make "noodles" out of beets and carrots, to use within the rolls.

1 serving soba or rice noodles (about 1 cup), cooked and
    drained

1 tablespoon toasted sesame oil

2 tablespoons black sesame seeds

1 cup pea shoots or sunflower sprouts, or 4–5 leaves of
    green leaf lettuce

10 ounces cooked chicken (leftovers from a roasted chicken
    or another meal), cut into strips

1 medium cucumber, peeled, seeds removed, and julienned

1 medium carrot, peeled and julienned

1 yellow bell pepper, seeded and julienned

4 large rounds (9 inches in diameter) rice paper wrappers

1 bunch cilantro, leaves only

½ cup fresh mint leaves

Garlic Hot and Sweet Dipping Sauce

½ cup water

¼ cup raw honey

2 tablespoons minced garlic

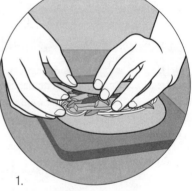

1.

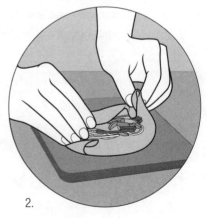

2.

1 tablespoon minced shallot

½ cup brown rice vinegar

1 tablespoon chopped cilantro

1 tablespoon red pepper flakes or chili sauce

sea salt

PREPARATION

Spring Rolls

Cook soba or rice noodles according to package instructions. Rinse in cool water and drain well. Toss with toasted sesame oil and set aside.

Have the chicken and vegetables ready on a large plate or in separate bowls. To make the rolls, work on top of a cutting board. 1. Soak a rice paper wrapper in a large bowl of lukewarm water for 30 seconds, until pliable. Shake off excess water and place on cutting board. Sprinkle with sesame seeds. 2. On the bottom one-third of the wrapper and about ¾ inch from the edge, place some sprouts or 1 leaf of lettuce, followed by a small band of noodles, a couple of strips of chicken, cucumber, carrot, bell pepper, and a few leaves of cilantro and mint.

3. Fold the bottom edge of the wrapper over the filling. Fold in the left and right edges and continue to roll up remaining wrapper tightly, forming a log. 4. Finish with the seam side down. Place on plate or platter. Make remaining rolls using all ingredients.

3.

Sauce

Bring ½ cup water to boil and add honey. Remove from heat and, whisking, dissolve honey. Add garlic and shallots; let cool. Add vinegar, cilantro, red pepper, and pinch of salt. Adjust seasonings as desired.

VARIATION

The peanut sauce from the soba noodles (page 169) is also delicious with the rolls.

4.

Spiced Sweet Potato "Risotto" with Chicken and Kale

SERVES 2

1½ cups chicken stock, vegetable stock, or water

3 tablespoons olive oil

1 pound boneless, skinless chicken breasts, cut into chunks

sea salt

1 tablespoon butter

½ cup diced onion

2 cups sweet potatoes, peeled and cut into medium chunks (about 3 cups)

1 tablespoon minced fresh gingerroot

2 cups green or red kale, torn into pieces

½ cup grated raw cheese

PREPARATION

Place stock or water in a pot on stove to warm.

Heat a skillet over medium-high heat until hot. Add 2 tablespoons of the olive oil and swirl to coat bottom of pan. Add chicken and a pinch of salt. Sauté 5 minutes, until chicken pieces have slightly browned. Remove chicken from pan with a slotted spoon and reserve on plate.

Add remaining 1 tablespoon of olive oil and 1 tablespoon of butter to pan. When foam from butter subsides, add onion and sauté for 3 minutes or until translucent. Add sweet potato, gingerroot, and a pinch of salt.

Sauté sweet potato for 3–5 minutes, until browned. Add ¼ cup of stock and stir while scraping brown bits from pan. When almost all liquid is gone, add another ¼ cup of stock. Continue to add liquid after the previous addition has evaporated until sweet potato is almost tender. With the last addition of liquid, add the cooked chicken, stirring together.

Cook until sweet potato has a little bite but is not mushy, about 12 minutes. Remove from heat, add kale, and mix well. Top with cheese and serve.

Stuffed Roasted Acorn Squash with Toasted Kasha, Greens, and Smoked Duck Breast

SERVES 1

1 medium-sized acorn squash

1 tablespoon olive oil

½ teaspoon ground cumin

½ teaspoon ground coriander

sea salt

½ bunch kale, sliced (about 2 loosely packed cups)

½ cup cooked kasha (buckwheat groats) or other grain

1 8-ounce smoked duck breast, cubed, fat removed

1 tablespoon hempseed oil

1 tablespoon sesame seeds

PREPARATION

Preheat oven to 425 degrees.

Cut off top of squash, about ¼ to ½ inch, and remove seeds. Slice a thin piece off the bottom so it will stand upright in pan. Rub inside of squash with olive oil, cumin, coriander, and a pinch of salt. Place in glass baking dish filled with ½ inch of water. Place dish in middle of oven. Cook 35–45 minutes, until fork-tender. When squash is done, remove dish from oven and transfer the squash to a serving plate.

Prepare kasha. When done, mix with kale while still hot. If using leftover kasha, place in a colander with kale, and place colander in sink. Bring ½ cup of water to boil and gently pour over kale and kasha. Transfer kale and kasha to a mixing bowl. Add duck, hempseed oil, sesame seeds, and a pinch of salt. Mix together, taste for seasoning, and spoon into squash. Serve.

Turkey Burgers

MAKES 4 BURGERS

Turkey burgers are a nice change from traditional beef burgers. Cooked correctly, they're just as moist and satisfying, and the possibilities are endless when it comes to toppings, sauces, and seasonings. For my recipe, the addition of chicken livers keeps the patty moist and adds a nice richness along with some great nutrients.

1 egg, lightly beaten
2 tablespoons chopped fresh sage leaves
1 tablespoon chopped fresh parsley
½ cup grated raw cheese
2 tablespoons sunflower seeds
sea salt
¼ pound chicken livers, chopped (optional)
1 pound ground turkey
½ cup cooked quinoa
1 tablespoon olive oil

PREPARATION

In a medium-sized mixing bowl, beat the egg. Add sage, parsley, cheese, sunflower seeds, and a pinch of salt; mix thoroughly. If using chicken livers, remove the veins and chop finely. Add to egg mixture along with ground turkey and quinoa. Using your hands, incorporate everything into the turkey, but don't overmix. Form 4–6 patties and lightly coat with olive oil. Set aside.

To Bake
Preheat oven to 375 degrees. Place burgers on a parchment-lined sheet pan and cook until done, about 10 minutes, flipping halfway through.

To Grill
Grill burgers over medium-high heat 3–4 minutes on each side, or until desired doneness is reached.

To Fry

Heat a nonstick skillet or pan with a swirl of olive oil over medium-high heat and cook burgers 3–4 minutes on each side.

GOOD ACCOMPANIMENTS

- Sprouted burger buns
- Grilled onions
- Sliced tomato
- Fresh mayonnaise (page 192)
- Sundried Tomato Spread (page 133)

MEAT

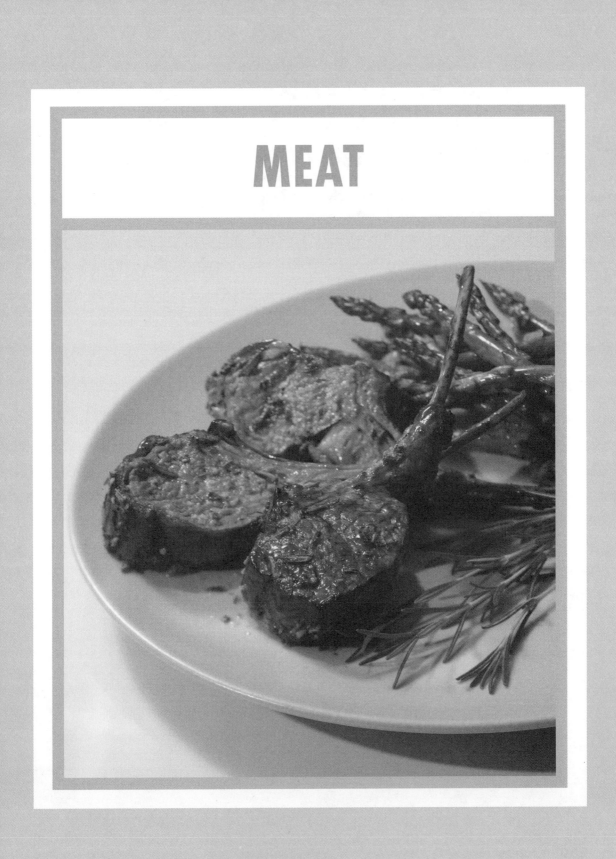

Broiled Lamb Rib Chops and Roasted Asparagus

SERVES 2

For Lamb

4 garlic cloves, peeled

1 bunch fresh rosemary, leaves removed and stems discarded

1 bunch fresh mint leaves

½ cup olive oil

juice of ½ lemon

sea salt and pepper

1 rack lamb rib chops, frenched* and trimmed (ask your butcher to do this for you)

For Asparagus

1 pound medium asparagus, root ends trimmed by 1 inch

1 tablespoon olive oil

1 tablespoon minced shallot

sea salt and freshly ground black pepper

¼ cup grated raw cheese

PREPARATION

Place garlic in food processor and finely mince. Scrape down the sides of the bowl with a rubber scraper and add rosemary, mint, and 2 tablespoons of the olive oil. Pulse until smooth. Add lemon juice. With processor running, remove the smaller lid and slowly add remaining olive oil in a thin stream until you have a nice, smooth paste. Add salt and pepper to taste.

Coat ribs with 75 percent of herb sauce. Marinate at least 2 hours, or overnight if possible.

Shortly before you plan to broil the ribs, toss asparagus with 1 tablespoon olive oil, shallots, and salt and pepper to taste. Place in a small baking dish and set aside.

*"Frenching" is cutting the meat away from the end of the chop so that part of the bone is exposed.

Preheat broiler and place oven rack 6 inches from flame or heat element.

Place ribs on broiler pan and cook 3–4 minutes on each side for medium rare. Cook the asparagus alongside the ribs under the broiler for the second 3–4 minutes, making sure not to overcook (the asparagus should have a slight bite or crunch).

Remove the lamb and the asparagus from the oven. Let the lamb rest a minute and then toss with remaining herb sauce. Top asparagus with cheese and serve.

Braised Pork Chop

SERVES 1

1 tablespoon olive oil

1 center-cut, bone-in pork chop, ¼ to ½ inch thick

sea salt

1 small onion, sliced thinly

1½ cups fresh, diced Roma tomatoes, juices included

1 tablespoon fresh thyme (or 1 teaspoon dried thyme)

1 tablespoon fresh oregano (or 1 teaspoon dried oregano)

¼ teaspoon red pepper flakes

½ cup freshly grated raw cheese

PREPARATION

Heat sauté pan over medium-high heat and add olive oil to pan. Let it get fairly hot, to where the oil seems to be shimmering.

Sprinkle the chop liberally with salt on both sides and place in pan. Immediately shake the pan slightly to prevent the chop from sticking; cook 5 minutes. Flip, add the sliced onions around the chop, and cook another 5 minutes. Add the tomatoes and a pinch of salt and cook for 3 minutes, or until the tomatoes break down slightly into a sauce.

Add the thyme, oregano, and red pepper and cover. Open the vent in the lid if there is one; otherwise, leave the lid slightly askew so steam can escape. Reduce the heat to medium-low and simmer 15–25 minutes, until chop is done. If liquid reduces too much, add water ¼ cup at a time.

To check doneness, if using an instant-read thermometer, aim for 135 degrees so the chop doesn't overcook. Another way to test if you're more experienced in handling meat or poultry is to press down on the chop. If you feel a slight springy resistance, you're good to go.

Top with freshly grated raw cheese.

- Polenta
- Pasta
- Salad
- Fresh or sautéed chard and kale; if you are preparing pasta, place chard or kale in the colander and drain the pasta over it for heat and flavor.

VARIATION

Chicken is an easy substitute for the pork. Follow the instructions for Pan-Roasted Chicken (page 221), but instead of placing chicken in oven, add 1½ cups fresh, chopped Roma tomatoes with a pinch of salt. Simmer in pan uncovered 15–20 minutes (a splatter shield is helpful), adding water to the pan as necessary.

Slow-Roasted Pork

SERVES 4–6

This dish is not quick to make, but it is very easy to prepare and can provide meat for a number of other meals during the week, or can be frozen for later use. The finished roast can be used in sandwiches, burritos, spring rolls, or fresh tomato sauce, with polenta, or with some grains and steamed veggies. When you divide the number of meals you can get into the time it takes to make, the proposition becomes very reasonable. I will make this about once a month on a Sunday when I am taking the time to prepare some dehydrated seeds and nuts, energy bars, food components for the week, or other snacks.

1 3- 4-pound bone-in pork shoulder (also called Boston butt or pork shoulder blade
    roast) with skin on, if possible
1 tablespoon olive oil
2 tablespoons minced garlic
1 tablespoon minced fresh gingerroot (optional)
sea salt
freshly ground black pepper

PREPARATION

Preheat oven to 475 degrees.

If you purchase a shoulder with the skin on, take a sharp knife and make small crisscrosses in it while trying not to reveal the meat underneath.

Either mix together with a fork, or blend using a small food processor, the olive oil, garlic, gingerroot, and pinch of salt and pepper into a paste. Rub all over the meat and into the grooves of the skin.

Place in large metal roasting pan with skin side up and put in oven on middle or lower rack. Roast for 25–30 minutes, until the top is golden brown. Reduce heat to 250 degrees and cook for 3–4 hours, until a meat thermometer placed into the thickest part reads 155–160 degrees and the meat is falling off the bone.

Remove from oven and let rest on cutting board for 20 minutes before serving.

Meanwhile, make a pan sauce: Pour off excess fat (which can be reserved for roasting potatoes) and place roasting pan on stove on medium-high heat. Add ½ cup water and bring to boil while scraping browned bits off of bottom using a wooden spoon.

GOOD ACCOMPANIMENTS

- Place chopped yams in pan for the last 45 minutes of cooking.
- Spring Rolls (page 222)
- Fresh polenta (page 158)
- Daily Antipasto (page 120)
- Grains

VARIATIONS

- Use the island rub (see page 196) for the pork.
- Give it an Asian flavor using a mixture of ½ cup tamari, 1 tablespoon sesame oil, 1 tablespoon honey, 1 tablespoon minced gingerroot, 3 cloves of minced garlic, 1 tablespoon fish sauce, and ½ bunch chopped cilantro.

Porky Reuben with Kraut, Cheddar, and Mustard

SERVES 1

The spice mixture adds a sweet, floral contrast to the sauerkraut and cheddar and makes this sandwich a global excursion for the palate. To prevent the rub from burning, it is best to prepare this in the oven.

1 teaspoon ground cumin (optional)
1 teaspoon ground coriander (optional)
½ teaspoon ground cloves (optional)
½ teaspoon ground ginger (optional)
sea salt
1 tablespoon olive oil
1 center-cut pork chop, about ¼–½ inch thick
sprouted bread roll, bun, or tortilla
prepared stone-ground brown mustard
3–4 slices raw cheddar cheese
½ cup raw sauerkraut (see recipe, page 145)

PREPARATION

Bring grill to high heat or preheat oven to 400 degrees.

If using spice mix, blend all together in small bowl along with a pinch of salt. Rub olive oil on both sides of chop and then dust with spice mixture. Place on grill and cook 7–9 minutes on each side, or place in baking dish and cook in oven for 12–15 minutes. The cooking time will vary depending on thickness.

Remove from heat and let rest for 2–3 minutes. Lightly toast sprouted bread roll, bun, or tortilla and spread with mustard. Cut meat off of bone and place on bread. Top with cheese and sauerkraut.

VARIATIONS

- Use Oven-Roasted or Pan-Roasted Chicken (pages 214 and 221)
- Use Slow-Roasted Pork (page 234)

DESSERTS

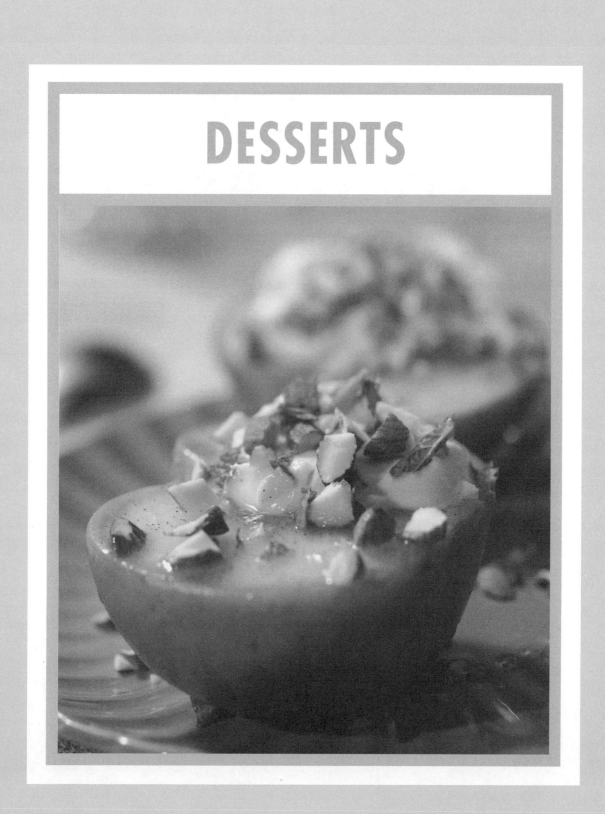

Baked Apples

SERVES 1

Nothing says fall quite like the best apples of the season. These baked treats make a fantastic breakfast, hearty snack, or even better dessert. To top it off, your whole kitchen will smell heavenly in minutes.

1 large apple (Gala, Empire, or Granny Smith all work well), cut in half and cored

1 teaspoon almond, coconut, or sesame oil

1 teaspoon raw apple cider vinegar

1 tablespoon maple syrup, raw honey, or agave nectar

¼ cup raisins (dark or golden)

¼ cup crushed raw walnuts, almonds, or cashews

2 tablespoons hemp seeds, sunflower seeds, or pumpkin seeds

1 tablespoon grated raw cheese or fresh, raw goat cheese

1 tablespoon chopped fresh mint leaves

sea salt

PREPARATION

Rub the apple halves with oil and place flesh side down on small sheet pan in 200-degree oven (a toaster oven works great here). Bake for 15–20 minutes, until warmed almost all the way through.

While apple is baking, toss the rest of the ingredients together in a small bowl and mix thoroughly. Once apple is done, top warm apple with mixture.

GOOD ACCOMPANIMENTS

- Salad
- Sprouted bread of your choice
- Quinoa
- Kasha (buckwheat groats)
- Couscous

Cashew Candy

MAKES 7 CUPS

This crunchy, healthful candy can be prepared using a dehydrator or a standard oven.

5 cups raw cashews, soaked 1–2 hours in water

2 cups dried, unsweetened mango pieces, diced

¼ cup shredded unsweetened coconut

½ cup brown rice syrup

¼ cup fresh lime juice

2 tablespoons black sesame seeds

2 tablespoons hemp seeds

sea salt

PREPARATION

Drain cashews well after soaking and place in mixing bowl. Toss with remaining ingredients, making sure that the nuts and fruit are evenly coated.

For dehydrator: Spread nut mixture on Teflex-lined tray and dehydrate at 115 degrees until dry.

For oven: Line a sheet tray with parchment paper and spread with nut mixture. Place tray in oven set on warm (or the lowest possible setting) and leave in oven all day or overnight, until dry. Store any leftovers in an airtight container for up to 1 month.

Ginger Date Coconut Chews

MAKES 12–16 CHEWS

These chews are a dessert and an energy snack at the same time. They are great after a meal or just to pop in your mouth when looking for a sweet pick-me-up.

2 cups fresh dates, pitted
1 tablespoon raw agave nectar
¾ cup plus 3 tablespoons shredded unsweetened coconut (medium shred)
¼ cup hemp seeds
2–3 tablespoons minced fresh gingerroot
seeds from ½ vanilla bean*
sea salt

PREPARATION

Place pitted dates and agave nectar in food processor. Pulse until just beyond chopped but before it becomes a sticky paste. Be careful not to heat the dates; stop the processor and allow to cool if this starts to happen.

Remove from processor and place in bowl with ¾ cup of the coconut, hemp seeds, gingerroot, vanilla bean seeds, and salt. Combine all of the ingredients thoroughly. Using a tablespoon, scoop out mixture and form into balls. Add the 3 tablespoons of coconut to the empty mixing bowl and toss in the date chews to coat. Store in airtight container in fridge.

*Split the bean open and scrape the small seeds from the sides using a paring knife.

VARIATION

For a chocolatey version, add ¼ cup cocoa or raw cacao powder to coconut mixture.

How to harvest vanilla caviar

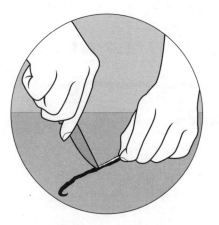

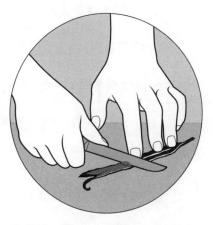

1. With a sharp paring knife, slice vanilla bean in half lengthwise.

2. Holding flat edge of blade against flesh, scrape bean in a smooth, fluid motion, collecting the seeds.

Grilled or Baked Peaches with Ginger Butter or Maple Crème Fraîche

SERVES 2

You can choose between the ginger butter or maple crème fraîche to top these delightful baked peaches, or go all out and use both.

2 large fresh peaches

1 tablespoon pure maple sugar

2 tablespoons almond oil or coconut oil

½ vanilla bean, split

1 tablespoon lemon juice

2 tablespoons chopped fresh mint leaves

2 tablespoons chopped raw almonds or cashews (can be sprouted)

Ginger-Butter Topping

2 tablespoons butter, softened (optional)

1 tablespoon minced fresh gingerroot

Crème Fraîche or Goat Cheese Topping

½ cup crème fraîche or fresh raw goat cheese

3 tablespoons pure maple syrup

PREPARATION

Start grill or heat oven to 400 degrees.

Slice peaches in half and remove pits. Combine maple sugar, oil, vanilla bean seeds (the interior of the bean), and lemon juice in a bowl. Add peach halves and, using hands or a wooden spoon, gently coat them with mixture.

For ginger-butter topping, mix softened butter (room temperature) with gingerroot. Set aside.

For crème fraîche or goat cheese topping, mix your choice with maple syrup. Set aside.

To Bake

Remove peaches from bowl and set facedown in baking dish. Bake 5–7 minutes, until warmed and just caramelizing on the bottom.

To Grill

Remove peaches from bowl and set facedown on grate. Grill 3–5 minutes, until just softened, with golden grill marks. Turn over and grill 3 more minutes.

Remove peaches from heat. Add 1 teaspoon butter in center, or top with 1–2 tablespoons crème fraîche or goat cheese. Sprinkle with mint and almonds. Serve warm.

Macaroons

MAKES ABOUT 28

I make these macaroons in a tablespoon size so that I can have 1 or 2 at a time. They are easy to prepare, store well, can be frozen, and disappear very quickly. As a bonus, with coconut and egg whites as main ingredients they are super-healthy pre- and post-training snacks.

2½ cups shredded, dried, unsweetened coconut (medium shred)
½ cup pure maple sugar
sea salt
2 egg whites
1 teaspoon vanilla extract or almond extract

PREPARATION

Preheat oven to 350 degrees.

Combine coconut, sugar, and sea salt in a bowl. Add egg whites and extract and mix well, making sure the mixture is wet (depending upon moisture of coconut and size of eggs, an additional egg white may be needed). Line an oven tray with parchment paper. Scoop mixture with a tablespoon; pack the mixture into the spoon, then slide onto tray, leaving space between cookies. Bake 15–20 minutes, until macaroons turn light golden brown. Cool and store in airtight container.

VARIATIONS

- Add 1 tablespoon dried lavender to add a complementary flavor to the coconut.
- Add 1 cup non-alkalized cocoa or raw cacao powder for a chocolate taste.
- For a raw version, use recipe as above, except omit egg whites, replace maple sugar with ½ cup maple syrup, and add ½ cup melted coconut butter. Mix ingredients and portion the same way. Place in dehydrator on Teflex sheets at 115 degrees until dried.

Maple Walnuts

MAKES 4 CUPS

I love this mixture as a snack, a quick pick-me-up, a topping for sorbet or ice cream, or even mixed with quinoa or couscous. This recipe can be prepared in an oven or a dehydrator.

4 cups raw walnuts, soaked 1–2 hours in water
½ cup pure maple syrup
1 cup diced crystallized ginger
1 cup diced, dried unsweetened papaya
3 tablespoons lime juice
1 tablespoon red pepper flakes (optional)
pinch of sea salt

PREPARATION

Drain walnuts well and place in mixing bowl. Toss with remaining ingredients, making sure that everything is evenly coated.

To bake, set oven on warm or the lowest possible setting. Line a sheet tray with parchment paper and spread nut mixture evenly on top. Place tray in oven and leave all day or overnight, until dry.

If using a dehydrator, spread nut mixture onto Teflex-lined trays and dehydrate at 115 degrees until dry.

Store in airtight container.

SNACKS

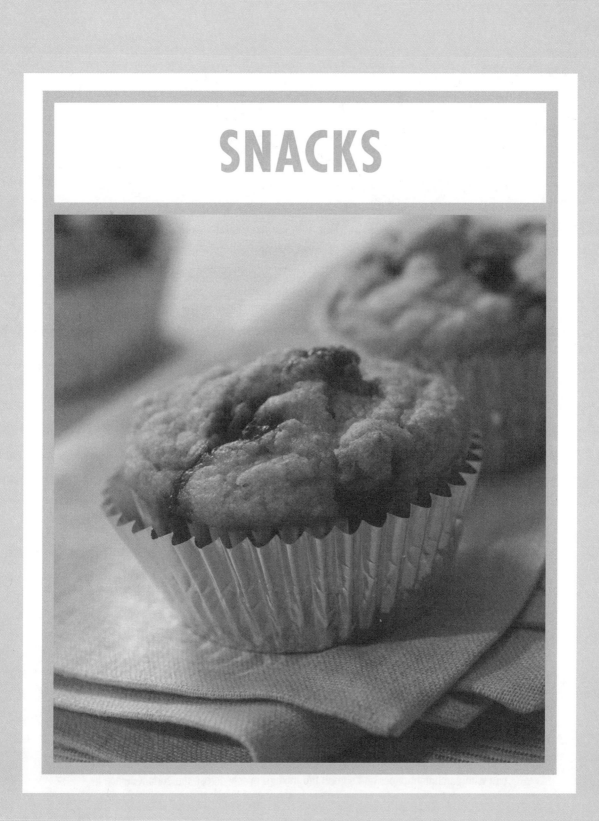

Power Granola

Granola is one of those things better made at home. Store-bought versions are usually packed with unnecessary refined sugar, corn syrup, and other unwanted ingredients. But when nuts, seeds, and dried fruit are used, the nutritional benefits of good, homemade granola are boundless.

This is a great food for athletes. It is very convenient and packed with goodness, from the fats in the nuts to the hemp seeds for protein and omegas, the goji berries for antioxidants, and the oats for carbs. You may use an oven or a dehydrator to prepare the granola.

Base Mixture

5 cups whole rolled oats

¼ cup coconut oil

2 teaspoons vanilla extract or almond extract

¼ cup pure maple syrup

3 teaspoons ground cinnamon

sea salt

Additions

I use all of the following, but feel free to pick and choose:

½ cup raw almonds

½ cup hemp seeds

½ cup raw pumpkin seeds or sunflower seeds

½ cup raw groats (sprouted buckwheat)

½ cup raw coconut flakes*

1 cup dried goji berries, blueberries, or raisins

PREPARATION

Preheat oven to 250 degrees.

In a large bowl, combine all the ingredients listed in the base mixture. Line a large sheet pan with parchment paper and spread the mixture evenly across the surface. Place in oven and stir every 7–10 minutes until desired doneness is reached. A light golden color should appear after about 20–25 minutes, but your nose is also a great way to tell if the mixture is done. Then add your choice of extras.

If using a dehydrator, mix all of the base ingredients together and dehydrate about 12–15 hours at 115 degrees. Then add your choice of extras.

GOOD ACCOMPANIMENTS

- Fresh fruit
- Raw milk
- Yogurt
- Grilled fruit

VARIATION

For a completely raw, trail-mix-like version, simply leave out the rolled outs and coconut oil and mix the rest of the ingredients together.

*Raw coconut flakes are dried at low temperature to retain their nutrients.

Morning Muffins

MAKES 12–16 MUFFINS

I am often pressed for time in the mornings, what with walking the dogs, getting my day together, and thinking about my training sessions. Making time to eat and thinking about what to eat can add stress to all of that, especially if my stomach is rumbling and I am worried about being fueled for a morning swim or run, or making a yoga class. Having something on the counter that I can trust, that is a quick grab, and that alleviates my worries goes a long way in setting the tone for the day.

These muffins combine simple and complex carbs that help jump-start the metabolism and provide some longer-lasting fuel to give you energy to start your workout or workday. Quickly warm them up and add some coconut butter, your favorite jam, or a bit of nut butter, and you are out the door!

Note that you can make a couple of batches at once and freeze some for later use.

1½ cups yellow cornmeal

1½ cups buckwheat flour, spelt flour, or quinoa flour

1 tablespoon baking powder (be sure to use non-aluminum)

sea salt

1 cup fresh or frozen blueberries

¼ cup pure maple syrup

1 tablespoon coconut oil

1 large egg

2 cups buttermilk, milk, yogurt, or water mixed with 1 heaping tablespoon almond, walnut, or cashew butter

1 teaspoon vanilla extract or almond extract

Preheat oven to 400 degrees.

In a large mixing bowl, combine cornmeal, flour, baking powder, and a dash of salt. Toss blueberries into dry mixture, evenly coating them (this will help prevent clumping when you add the wet mixture).

In a separate bowl, combine maple syrup, oil, egg, buttermilk, and extract. Quickly fold into dry mixture using as few strokes as possible to prevent overmixing, which will make the muffins tough.

Use a ceramic muffin pan or line a metal muffin pan with paper cups (a silicone pan will work as well) and evenly distribute the muffin mixture into each cup. Do not fill; leave room for rising during baking.

Place muffins on center oven rack. Bake 25–30 minutes, or until golden brown and a toothpick comes out clean (no wet batter clinging to it) when inserted and removed.

Remove pan from oven and let cool 5 minutes. Remove muffins and let finish cooling on wire rack or counter.

Muffins can be frozen up to 2 months or stored in an airtight container up to a week.

VARIATION

Soak flour in buttermilk for 12–24 hours. The muffins will rise better, and soaking will add a quick ferment to the process.

How to measure flour

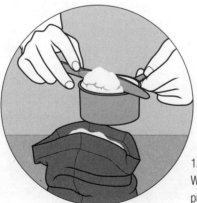

1. Scoop flour without packing in. With flat edge of knife, level flour by pushing excess off in a fluid motion.

Morning Quinoa

SERVES 2

A great alternative to oatmeal or granola, this morning grain is full of the good carbs you need to get energy pumping and get you ready to face the day. Add dried fruit and other seeds as your taste buds desire.

See the instructions for cooking quinoa on page 174.

1 cup cooked quinoa

¼ cup almonds, chopped

¼ cup raisins

¼ cup sunflower seeds

½ pear or apple, diced (dried papaya and apricots work very well also)

1 tablespoon hemp seeds

1 tablespoon raw pumpkin seed oil

1 tablespoon raw honey, pure maple syrup, or agave nectar

¼ cup nut milk, seed milk, or raw dairy milk (optional)

PREPARATION

If the quinoa has been refrigerated, let it come to room temperature. Mix the dry ingredients into the quinoa along with oil and then add the sweetener. If you are using a milk, either warm slightly first or add cold, depending on whether you want a warm or cold breakfast.

Three Nut Butter Variations with Fruit

SERVES 1

Revisiting your favorite childhood snacks is a great way to reminisce and satisfy a craving. Luckily for many (including myself), cut-up apples with honey and peanut butter were a popular snack when we were young, and they can still be a healthy one for adults. Any of these mixes can be tucked into a small airtight container and thrown in a bag with an apple, pear, banana, or whatever you fancy for a quick pre- or post-training snack.

Sweet

2 tablespoons raw almond butter or cashew butter

1 tablespoon raw honey or pure maple syrup

1 tablespoon raw coconut butter

Spicy

2 tablespoons raw walnut butter

1 tablespoon raw honey

½ teaspoon cayenne pepper

Tropical

1 tablespoon raw almond butter

2 tablespoons raw honey

1 tablespoon shredded unsweetened coconut

1 teaspoon lime juice

PREPARATION FOR ALL THREE VERSIONS

Mix ingredients together in small bowl until combined.

VARIATION

Place a bowl of grapes (mixed colors a plus!) in the freezer for 3–5 minutes and then toss with the tropical mixture for a quick dessert (serve in a martini glass). Also good with fresh sliced mango.

Popcorn

Popcorn is nutritious, full of fiber, and easy to make, all rolled up in fun! This was my energy snack while traveling in India and Nepal, where it was cooked kettle-style. You can use a popcorn machine if you have one, but there's no need to buy an appliance when popcorn is so easy to make on top of the stove.

½ cup popcorn kernels
2 tablespoons coconut oil
½ tablespoon olive oil

PREPARATION

Heat a large pot with a well-fitting lid over high heat. After a few minutes, add oil and turn down heat to medium-low. Swirl to coat bottom of pan and then add popcorn. Toss popcorn to coat with oil and then top with lid. Continue cooking while shaking back and forth as the kernels pop to keep the popcorn from burning. Once the popping has subsided, turn heat to low and continue shaking for 1 minute. Turn off the heat, remove from burner, and allow residual heat to pop any remaining kernels. Once finished, transfer to a bowl and eat, or keep warm in pot while you prepare a topping.

VARIATIONS

- Sea salt
- Grated raw cheese
- Ginger butter: Add 1 tablespoon minced gingerroot to 2 tablespoons butter, heat together, and pour melted mixture over popcorn.
- Maple syrup
- Cocoa butter: Add 1 tablespoon non-aluminum cocoa powder to 2 tablespoons butter, heat together, and pour melted mixture over popcorn.
- Cajun corn: Mix together 1 tablespoon smoked paprika, ½ tablespoon ground cayenne, 1 teaspoon sea salt, and 1 teaspoon ground mustard. Toss popcorn with 3 tablespoons melted butter, then dust with spice mix.
- Apple-cinnamon: Mix 1 tablespoon ground cinnamon, 1 teaspoon ground nutmeg, 1 teaspoon ground cloves, and ½ cup chopped dried apples. Melt 3 tablespoons

butter with 1 tablespoon minced gingerroot. Toss ginger butter with popcorn and then dust with spice mixture.

- Use a spray bottle to mist popcorn with Nama Shoyu or other soy sauce.
- Toss hot popcorn with curry powder and ground turmeric for an Indian-scented spicy mix.

Omega Hummus with Bee Pollen

SERVES 4–6

This is a great post-workout snack or meal, not only because it is easy to prepare but also because it has an optimum protein-to-carb ratio and all the ingredients to regulate insulin. Chickpeas, in fact, provide more receptors for insulin, thus allowing your body to replenish its glycogen stores quickly and efficiently. Bee pollen adds B vitamins for recovery as well as nutrients to help support the immune system. For myself and my clients, this is a snack to have in the fridge at all times.

2 cloves garlic, peeled

1 tablespoon bee pollen

1 cup cooked or sprouted chickpeas (garbanzo beans), drained, outer skins removed

1½ tablespoons raw sesame tahini

¼ cup olive oil

¼ cup flaxseed oil or sunflower oil

¼ cup hempseed oil

juice of 1 lemon

sea salt

PREPARATION

In the bowl of a food processor, finely mince the garlic and bee pollen. Add chickpeas and remaining ingredients and pulse until smooth. Taste for seasoning and add salt as needed. Refrigerate in an airtight container up to 2 weeks.

GOOD ACCOMPANIMENTS

- Raw veggies
- Whole-grain crackers
- Sandwiches

7

Resources

Kitchen Equipment

Listed below are the kitchen items that I find indispensable. They will simplify your cooking, provide options for a variety of eating and preparation habits, and keep you healthy. It is important to be just as smart and health-conscious when buying kitchen equipment as when buying food, especially those items that will have direct contact with food. Food can absorb harmful chemicals when heated in nonstick cookware, for example. Plastic storage containers can also leach chemicals, especially over time and extended use (see "The Right Gear to Carry Your Fuel" in Chapter 5 for more information). Limiting the purchase and use of appliances is best for the environment, your cupboard space, and your electric bills. When you shop for appliances, try to find those that are multiuse and well built. Cheap blenders, for example, are a dime a dozen; buying a high-quality blender will guarantee that it will last a long time. This is true of cookware as well. Buy the things that you are going to realistically use. Split the cost of a large or expensive item, such as a dehydrator, with a friend who shares your interest in healthy cooking.

High-quality water filter (countertop, under-sink, or
   whole-house)

Vita-mix blender

Harsch fermenting crock

Excalibur dehydrator

Food processor or multiuse hand mixer

Stainless-steel, clay, or ceramic cookware, including
   braising pot, oval roaster for fish, Dutch oven,
   large fry pan, stockpot with lid, sauté pan with lid,
   saucepans with lids, and large baking pan

Bamboo steamer set

Bamboo cutting board or one made from sustainable
   wood (look for a label indication)

Bamboo or wooden spoons

Ceramic muffin pan

Pizza stone for bread making

Glass food storage containers for both cooked and
   dry foods

Mason jars for sprouting and food storage

Teapot

Mandoline or Benriner

Spiralizer (spiral slicer)

Grain mill

Coffee grinder and French press coffeemaker

Glass mixing bowls

Large colander

High-quality knife set

Stainless-steel hand tools, including tongs,
   long-handled spoons, fish spatula, whisk,
   measuring cups and spoons, and cheese grater

Kitchen shears

Compost pail

Electric juicer (Breville is a good brand)

Reusable shopping bags (preferably made from
   recycled or organic materials)

Pots for growing herbs and vegetables

Solar oven

Kitchen Pantry and Fridge

The more food components you have on hand, the easier and more creative cooking can be, especially when time is short. Buying items in bulk that have a long shelf life, such as grains and dried beans and fruits, helps to limit the number of shopping excursions you take and is cost-efficient. In my own pantry, everything is organic and, when suitable, raw and sprouted. I do not necessarily have all the following ingredients all of the time; this is a rotating list of items that I try to have on hand, along with any of the spreads and sauces from the "Recipes" chapter that I have made and stored in the fridge. Anything that I might consider buying in a can or jar I try to make myself.

All, or nearly all, of the ingredients below can be found in your local grocery store or supermarket, though you might need to poke around a bit to find them. See also the "Foods and Seed Sources" section if you cannot find what you are looking for in your neighborhood.

Oils and Vinegars

It is important to make sure that oils are virgin and cold-pressed or expeller-pressed.

Coconut oil

Flaxseed oil

Hempseed oil

Olive oil
Pumpkin seed oil
Sesame oil
Toasted sesame oil
Walnut oil

Apple cider vinegar
Balsamic vinegar
Brown rice vinegar
Coconut vinegar
Red wine vinegar
Rice wine vinegar
White wine or champagne vinegar

Sauces and Spreads
Agave nectar
Almond butter
Cashew butter
Coconut butter
Coconut milk
Fish sauce (nam pla)
Ghee (clarified butter)
Honey (raw)
Kimchi
Maple syrup
Mirin
Miso paste
Nama Shoyu soy sauce (a raw, unpasteurized,
    organic soy sauce)
Red and green curry paste
Sauerkraut
Tahini
Tamari
Walnut butter

Beans
Heirloom beans, such as black, yellow Indian woman,
    garbanzo, vaquero, tepary, and azuki
Sprouting seeds and beans, including mung, pea,
    pumpkin, sunflower, and sesame

Sprouted Seeds, Nuts, and Dried Fruit
Pumpkin seeds
Sunflower seeds

Almonds
Brazil nuts
Cashews
Walnuts

Apple
Coconut
Dates
Figs
Goji berries
Mango
Papaya
Pineapple

Seaweeds
Arame
Dulse (also available smoked)
Hijiki
Kombu
Nori
Wakame

Grains
Assorted soba noodles and pastas
Barley
Brown rice

Buckwheat groats (kasha)
Quinoa
Wild rice

"Super Foods"
Acerola powder
Activated barley powder
Bee pollen
Camu camu powder
Fermented cod liver oil
Freeze-dried organ extracts (heart, kidney, lungs,
    generally bovine; see source below)
Hemp protein powder
High-vitamin butter oil
Krill oil
Maca root powder
Pea powder
SunPower Greens
Whey protein powder

Spices
Almond extract
Arrowroot powder
Black peppercorns
Cinnamon powder
Coriander seed
Cumin seed
Curry powder
Hemp seed
Red pepper flakes
Sea salt
Turmeric
Vanilla bean
Vanilla extract
Wasabi powder

Miscellaneous
Bonito flakes
Cured olives
Heirloom popcorn

Informational Websites

Collaborative on Health
and the Environment
An online network that addresses growing concerns about the links between human health and environmental factors.
www.healthandenvironment.org

Organic Consumers Association (OCA)
The OCA deals with issues of food safety, industrial agriculture, genetic engineering, children's health, and corporate accountability, fair trade, and environmental sustainability.
www.organicconsumers.org

Physicians for Social Responsibility
A resource and watchdog group for the protection of health.
www.envirohealthaction.org

U.S. Department of Health
and Human Services
Health and safety information on household products.
http://householdproducts.nlm.nih.gov/index.htm

Weston A. Price Foundation
Named for the physician who pioneered nutrition studies, this nonprofit charity is dedicated to restoring nutrient-dense foods to the human diet through education, research, and activism.
www.westonaprice.org

Foods and Seed Sources

Baker Creek Heirloom Seeds
http://rareseeds.com

Dr. Ron's Ultra Pure (freeze-dried organs, fermented cod liver oil, traditional food supplements)
www.drrons.com

Earth Family Foods (raw and "super" foods)
www.earthfamilyfoods.com

Fermented Treasures (cultured food and beverage starter cultures)
www.fermentedtreasures.com

GEM Cultures (bread ferments, soy, and dairy cultures)
www.gemcultures.com

Gernot Katzer's Spice Pages (an encyclopedic resource of spices)
www.uni-graz.at/~katzer/engl

Gold Mine Natural Foods
www.goldminenaturalfoods.com

GoRaw (sprouted seeds, raw granola, and treats)
www.goraw.com

Green Pastures (beneficial oils)
www.greenpasture.org/community

Living Nutz (live organic foods)
www.livingnutz.com/index.html

Mercola.com (well-researched products, including krill oil, ceramic cookware, raw whey, and pea protein powder)
www.mercola.com

Mum's Sprouting Seeds (seeds and supplies)
www.sprouting.com

Organic Performance (SunPower Greens, carefully selected food and lifestyle goods)
www.organicperformance.com

Rancho Gordo (heirloom beans)
www.ranchogordo.com/index.htm

Seed Savers Exchange (heirloom seeds)
www.seedsavers.org

South River Miso Company
www.southrivermiso.com

SproutPeople (seeds and supplies)
www.sproutpeople.com

Victory Seeds (rare, open-pollinated,
and heirloom seeds)
www.victoryseeds.com

Wilderness Family Naturals ("super foods")
www.wildernessfamilynaturals.com

Household and Natural Products Sources
The Campaign for Safe Cosmetics
www.safecosmetics.org

Doulton USA (water filtration)
www.doultonusa.com

Earth Friendly Products (cleaning products)
www.ecos.com

Environmental Working Group
www.ewg.org

Natural Products Association
www.naturalproductsassoc.org

Seventh Generation (cleaning products)
www.seventhgeneration.com

Sun and Earth (cleaning products)
www.sunandearth.com

Tensui Water Perfection Systems
www.tensuiwater.com

Twist (cleaning supplies)
www.twist.com

Seasonal Food Availability and Farmers' Markets
Center for Urban Education
about Sustainable Agriculture
(seasonal food chart)
www.cuesa.org/index.php

Eat Well Guide (farmers' markets,
food stores, restaurants, and shops)
www.eatwellguide.org

Local Harvest (seasonal availability and
direct-from-farm purchase)
www.localharvest.org

National Sustainable Agriculture
Information Service (local food directory
and resource for information on sustainable
agriculture practices)
http://attra.ncat.org

Sustainable Table (seasonal availability
of food, farmers' markets, CSAs, and
sustainable food choices)
www.sustainabletable.org/home.php

Conversion Tables

Baking and Cooking Measurements

1 tablespoon	=	½ ounce	=	3 teaspoons
¼ cup	=	2 ounces	=	4 tablespoons
½ cup	=	4 ounces	=	8 tablespoons
¾ cup	=	6 ounces	=	12 tablespoons
1 cup	=	8 ounces	=	16 tablespoons
2 cups	=	1 pint	=	1 pound
1 pint	=	16 ounces	=	1 pound
2 pints	=	1 quart	=	4 cups
1 quart	=	4 cups	=	2 pounds
1 gallon	=	4 quarts	=	8 pounds
1 ounce	=	30 grams		
1 pound	=	16 ounces	=	454 grams
½ pound	=	8 ounces	=	225 grams
2.2 pounds	=	1 kilogram		

Oven Temperatures

Temperature	Fahrenheit	Celsius
very low	150°F	70°C
low	200°F	100°C
medium	350°F	180°C
hot	425°F	210°C
very hot or grill	500°F	260°C

Appendix

Genetically Modified Ingredients Overview

The following is a summary of the crops, foods, and food ingredients that have been genetically modified (GM) as of July 2007. The information comes from the Institute for Responsible Technology (http://www.responsibletechnology.org).

Currently Commercialized GM Crops in the United States

The number in parentheses represents the estimated percentage of the product that is genetically modified.

Soy (89%)
Cotton (83%)
Canola (75%)
Corn (61%)
Hawaiian papaya (more than 50%)

Other GM Sources

Dairy products from cows injected with rbGH

Food additives, enzymes, flavorings, and processing agents, including the sweetener aspartame (NutraSweet®) and rennet used to make hard cheeses

Honey and bee pollen that may have GM sources of pollen

Meat, eggs, and dairy products from animals that have eaten GM feed

Ingredients Derived from Soybeans

Soy flour, soy protein, soy isolates, soy isoflavones, soy lecithin, vegetable proteins, textured vegetable protein (TVP), tofu, tamari, tempeh, and soy protein supplements

Ingredients Derived from Corn

Corn flour, corn gluten, corn masa, cornstarch, corn syrup, cornmeal, and high-fructose corn syrup (HFCS)

Food Additives Derived from GM Sources

Ascorbic acid/ascorbate (vitamin C), cellulose, citric acid, cobalamin (vitamin B12), cyclodextrin, cystein, dextrin, dextrose, diacetyl, fructose (especially crystalline fructose), glucose, glutamate, glutamic acid, gluten, glycerides (mono- and diglycerides), glycerol, glycerine, glycine, hemicellulose, hydrogenated starch hydrolates, hydrolyzed vegetable protein or starch, inositol, invert sugar or inverse syrup (also may be listed as inversol or colorose), lactic acid, lactoflavin, lecithin, leucine, lysine, maltose, maltitol, maltodextrin, mannitol, methylcellulose, milo starch, modified food starch, monooleate, mono- and diglycerides, monosodium glutamate (MSG), oleic acid, phenylalanine, phytic acid, riboflavin (vitamin B2), sorbitol, stearic acid, threonine, tocopherol (vitamin E), trehalose, xanthan gum, and zein.

Foods That May Contain GM Ingredients

Alcohol
Baking powder (sometimes contains cornstarch)
Bread
Candy
Cereal
Chips
Chocolate
Confectioner's glaze
Confectioner's sugar (often contains cornstarch)
Cookies
Crackers
Enriched flour
Fried food
Frozen yogurt
Hamburgers
Hot dogs
Ice cream
Infant formula
Malt
Margarine
Mayonnaise
Meat substitutes
Pasta
Peanut butter
Powdered sugar
Protein powder
Salad dressing
Soy cheese
Soy sauce
Tamari
Tofu
Tomato sauce
Vanilla extract (sometimes contains corn syrup)
Veggie burgers
White vinegar

Nonfood Items That May Contain GM Ingredients

Bubble bath
Cosmetics
Detergents
Shampoo
Soaps

Notes

Chapter 1

1. Scott Jurek's website, www.scottjurek.com.

2. Speech given by Dave Scott at Silverman Full Distance Triathlon, November 2006.

3. United States Environmental Protection Agency, *Ag 101: Demographics,* 2009, www.epagov/oecaagct/ag101/demographics.html.

4. Donald R. Davis, "Declining Fruit and Vegetable Nutrient Composition: What Is the Evidence?" *Horticultural Science* 44, 1 (February 2009).

5. Rich Pirog and Andrew Benjamin, *Checking the Food Odometer: Comparing Food Miles for Local Versus Conventional Produce Sales to Iowa Institutions* (Ames, IA: Leopold Center for Sustainable Agriculture, 2003).

6. Charles Benbrook, Xin Zhao, Jaime Yáñez, Neal Davies, and Preston Andrews, "New Evidence Confirms the Nutritional Superiority of Plant-Based Organic Food," *State of Science Review,* March 2008. The Organic Center, www.organic-center.org.

7. Marion Nestle, *Safe Food* (Berkeley: University of California Press, 2003), 121.

8. Ibid., 126.

9. USDA, Economic Research Service, 2008, Table 52: High Fructose Corn Syrup: Estimated Number of Per Capita Calories Consumed Daily, by Calendar Year.

10. Jack Challem, "Fructose: Maybe Not So Natural . . . and Not So Safe," *Nutrition Reporter,* 1996, www.thenutritionreporter.com/fructose_dangers.html.

11. Edward Howell, *Enzyme Nutrition: The Food Enzyme Concept* (Wayne, NJ: Avery Publishing Group, 1985), 6.

12. Interview with Jeffery Boost, PAC, March 2009.

13. Ibid.

14. "The Intravenous Use of Coconut Water," *American Journal of Emergency Medicine* 18, 1 (January 2000): 108–111.

15. Press release, Wheat Foods Council, April 1, 2006.

Chapter 2

1. Dan Shapley, "Time to Stop Using Nerve Gas on Farms? Lawsuit Challenges Legality of WWII-Era Chemicals," April 8, 2008. The Daily Green online, www.thedailygreen.com/environmental-news/latest/pesticides-47040804.

2. Marion Nestle, *Safe Food* (Berkeley: University of California Press, 2003), 184.

3. *The World According to Monsanto,* documentary.

4. Consumers Union, "Are Organic Foods as Good as They're Grown?" December 15, 1997, Consumers Union Press Release.

5. Mary Jane Incorvia Mattina, William Iannucci-Berger, and Laure Dykas, "Chlordane Uptake and Its Translocation in Food Crops," *Journal of Agriculture and Food Chemicals* 48, 5 (2000): 1909–1915.

6. Chensheng Lu, Kathryn Toepel, Rene Irish, Richard A. Fenske, Dana B. Barr, and Roberto

Bravo, "Organic Diets Significantly Lower Children's Dietary Exposure to Organophosphorus Pesticides," *Environmental Health Perspectives* 114, 2 (February 2006): 261–263.

7. "The U.S. Ban on DDT: A Continuing Success Story," April 4, 2005, Environmental Defense Fund Online, www.edf.org.

8. Rick Relyea, "The Impact of Insecticides and Herbicides on the Biodiversity and Productivity of Aquatic Communities," *Journal of Ecological Applications* 15, 2 (April 2005): 618–627.

9. Cancer Prevention Coalition, "Monsanto's Hormonal Milk Poses Serious Risks of Breast Cancer, Besides Other Cancers, Warns Professor of Environmental Medicine at the University of Illinois School of Public Health." June 21, 1998, www.preventcancer.com; S. Rinaldi et al., "IGF-I, IGFBP-3 and Breast Cancer Risk in Women: The European Prospective Investigation into Cancer and Nutrition (EPIC)," *Endocrine Related Cancer* 13, 2 (June 2006): 593–605; Judith Perera, "Mad Cows, rBGH Hormones Related," *Albion Monitor,* December 8, 1996, www.albionmonitor.com.

10. "20 Questions on Genetically Modified Foods," World Health Organization, www.who.int/foodsafety/publications/biotech/20questions/en/.

11. *Federal Register* 57, 104 (1992): 22991.

12. Michael Pollan, "Playing God in the Garden," *New York Times*, October 25, 1998.

13. R. Schubbert, U. Hohlweg, D. Renz, and W. Doerfler, "On the Fate of Orally Ingested Foreign DNA in Mice: Chromosomal Association and Placental Transmission in the Fetus," *Molecules, Genes, and Genetics* 259 (1998): 569–576.

14. Jeffrey M. Smith, *Genetic Roulette: The Documented Health Risks of Genetically Engineered Foods* (White River Junction, VT: Chelsea Green, 2007).

15. Donald R. Davis, "Declining Fruit and Vegetable Nutrient Composition: What Is the Evidence?" *Horticultural Science* 44, 1 (February 2009): 15–19.

16. Virginia Worthington, "Nutritional Quality of Organic Versus Conventional Fruits, Vegetables, and Grains," *Journal of Alternative and Complementary Medicine* 7, 2 (2001): 161–173.

17. *Variations in Mineral Content in Vegetables,* Firman E. Baer Report from Rutgers University, 1984.

18. Interview with Jamie Mitchell, March 2009.

19. *Recent Growth Patterns in the U.S. Organic Foods Market,* Economic Research Service/USDA, 2000.

20. Interview with Terri Schneider, March 2009.

21. Interview with Mike Richter, April 2009.

22. Dan Benardot, *Nutrition for Serious Athletes* (Champaign, IL: Human Kinetics, 1999).

23. Based on personal experience.

24. Ying Wu, Aiko K. Perry, and Barbara P. Klein, "Vitamin C and Beta-Carotene in Fresh and Frozen Green Beans and Broccoli in a Simulated System," *Journal of Food Quality* 15, 2 (October 1991): 87–96.

25. Ying Wu, Aiko K. Perry, and Barbara P. Klein, "Vitamin C and Beta-carotene in Fresh and Frozen Green Beans and Broccoli in a Simulated System," Journal of Food Quality 15, 2 (1992): 87–96.

26. Interview with Sara Hanafin, April 2003.

27. "Globetrotting Food Will Travel Farther Than Ever This Thanksgiving," Worldwatch Institute, November 21, 2002, www.worldwatch.org.

28. Karen Page and Andrew Dornenburg, *Culinary Artistry* (New York: John Wiley & Sons, 1996), 28.

29. Geneen Roth, *When Food Is Love: Exploring the Relationship Between Eating and Intimacy* (New York: Penguin, 1991), 103.

30. Donald Reid, *The Tao of Health, Sex and Longevity: A Modern Practical Guide to the Ancient Way* (New York: Simon and Schuster, 1989), 80.

31. Stephen Harrod Buhner, *The Fasting Path: The Way to Spiritual, Physical, and Emotional Enlightenment* (New York: Avery, 2003), 62.

32. Interview with Bernd Heinrich, March 2009.

Chapter 3

1. Interview with Mike Richter, April 2009.

2. "Supermarket Facts: Industry Overview 2006," Food Market Institute, www.fmi.org/facts_figs/superfact.htm.

3. USFDA. IX. Appendix A: Definitions of Nutrient Content Claims. Guidance for Industry: A Food Labeling Guide. April 2008, www.fda.gov.

4. Marion Nestle, *Safe Food* (Berkeley: University of California Press, 2003), 78.

5. Ronald H. Schmidt and Gary E. Rodrick, *Food Safety Handbook* (New York: Wiley-IEEE, 2005), 611.

6. Ibid.

7. Emma Dorey, "Food for Life: Despite Increasing Evidence That Folic Acid Benefits Both Young and Old, the Food Fortification Debate Rages on in the UK," *Journal of Chemistry and Industry,* January 29, 2007.

8. Jeremy Elton Jacquot, "The Great Pacific Garbage Patch: Out of Sight, Out of Mind," February 7, 2008, www.treehugger.com/files/2008/02/great_pacific_garbage_patch.php;www.greatgarbagepatch.com.

9. Interview with Dr. John Ivy, March 2009.

10. Bernd Heinrich, *Racing the Antelope: What Animals Can Teach Us About Running and Life* (New York: HarperCollins, 2003), 208.

11. Amy Paturel and Brierley Wright, "How the Elite Eat: Four Top Athletes Share Their Winning Secrets to Healthy Eating," Eating Well, www.eatingwell.com/nutrition_health/nutrition_news_information/how_the_elite_eat?page.

Chapter 4

1. USFDA, Draft Guidance: Whole Grain Label Statements, February 17, 2006.

2. "U.S. Sales of Organic Food Jump 16 Percent in 2008," Flex News Online, June 5, 2009.

3. Virginia Worthington, "Nutritional Quality of Organic Versus Conventional Fruits, Vegetables, and Grains," *Journal of Alternative and Complementary Medicine* 7, 2 (2001): 161–173.

4. Interview with Dr. Thomas Cowan, March 2009.

5. Interview with Liz Applegate, May 2003.

6. "Controlling the Global Obesity Epidemic," no date listed, World Health Organization, www.who.int.

7. "Obesity and Overweight: Fact Sheet No. 311," September 2006, World Health Organization, www.who.int/mediacentre/factsheets/fs311/en/.

8. Cynthia L. Ogden, Margaret D. Carroll, Margaret A. McDowell, and Katherine M. Flegal, "Obesity Among Adults in the United States: No Statistically Significant Change Since 2003–2004," November 2007, National Center for Health Statistics, www.cdc.gov/nchs/.

9. NHANES Surveys (1976–1980 and 2003–2006), Trends in Childhood Obesity, Center for Disease Control, www.cdc.gov.

10. Yunsheng Ma et al., "Association Between Eating Patterns and Obesity in a Free-Living U.S. Adult Population," *American Journal of Epidemiology* 158 (2003): 85–92.

Chapter 5

1. John Ivy and Robert Portman, *The Performance Zone: Your Nutrition Action Plan for Greater Endurance and Sports Performance* (Laguna Beach, CA: Basic Health, 2004), 11.

2. Joseph Charles Maroon and Jeffrey W. Bost, "X-3 Fatty Acids (Fish Oil) as an Anti-inflammatory: An Alternative to Nonsteroidal Anti-inflammatory Drugs for Discogenic Pain," *Surgical Neurology* 65 (2006): 326–331.

3. Ron Schmid, *The Untold Story of Milk: The History, Politics, and Science of Nature's Perfect Food: Raw Milk from Pastured-Fed Cows* (Washington, DC: New Trends Publishing, 2009).

4. Peter J. Horvath, Colleen K. Eagen, Stacie D. Ryer-Calvin, and David R. Pendergast, "The Effects of Varying Dietary Fat on the Nutrient Intake in Male and Female Runners," *Journal of the American College of Nutrition* 19, 1 (2000): 42–51.

5. "Micronutrients," World Health Organization, www.who.int/nutrition/topics/micronutrients/en/.

6. Interview with Terry Graham, September 2004, along with other research.

7. Dan Benardot, *Nutrition for Serious Athletes* (Champaign, IL: Human Kinetics, 1999).

8. Mark Jenkins, "Caffeine and the Athlete," SportsMed Web Online, http://www.rice.edu/~jenky/sports/caffeine.html.

9. Sally Fallon and Mary G. Enig, *Nourishing Traditions: The Cookbook That Challenges Politically Correct Nutrition and the Diet Dictocrats* (Winona Lake, IN: New Trends Publishing, 1999), 285.

10. Interview with Dr. John Ivy, March 2009.

11. Interview with Terri Schneider, March 2009.

12. Interview with Dr. John Ivy, March 2009.

Chapter 6

1. Interview with Jamie Mitchell, April 2009.

2. Edward Howell, *Enzyme Nutrition: The Food Enzyme Concept* (Wayne, NJ: Avery Publishing, 1985).

3. David Wolfe, *The Sunfood Diet Success System* (San Diego, CA: Maul Brothers, 2006), 203.

4. Howell, *Enzyme Nutrition*, p. 120.

5. Dirk Matthys, Patrick Calders, Jean-Louis Pannier, and Wim Derave, "Effect of Branched-Chain Amino Acids (BCAA), Glucose, and Glucose Plus BCAA on Endurance Performance in Rats," *Medicine and Science in Sports and Exercise* 31, 4 (April 1999): 583–587; Alan Christianson, "Ergogenics for Endurance Athletes," *Nutrition Science News* (March 2000), www.newhope.com/nutritionsciencenews/NSN_backs/Mar_00/athletes.cfm.

6. John Ivy and Robert Portman, *The Performance Zone: Your Nutrition Action Plan for Greater Endurance* (Laguna Beach, CA: Basic Health Publications, 2004), p. 104.

Bibliography

Antonio, J., and J. Stout. *Supplements for Endurance Athletes.* Champaign, IL: Human Kinetics, 2002.

Aoi, W., Y. Naito, and T. Yoshikawa. "Exercise and Functional Foods." *Nutrition Journal* 5 (2006): 15.

Arcury, T. A., S. A. Quandt, and B. G. Mellen. "An Exploratory Analysis of Occupational Skin Disease Among Latino Migrant and Seasonal Farmworkers in North Carolina." *Journal of Agricultural Safety and Health* 9, 3: 221–232.

Benet, S. "Why They Live to Be 100, or Even Older, in Abkhasia: Faces in an Abkhasian Crowd." *New York Times Magazine,* December 26, 1971.

Berardi, J. M., E. E. Noreen, and P.W.R. Lemon. "Recovery from a Cycling Time Trial Is Enhanced with Carbohydrate-Protein Supplementation vs. Isoenergetic Carbohydrate Supplementation." *Journal of the International Society of Sports Nutrition* 5 (2008): 24.

Buhner, S. *Lost Language of Plants: The Ecological Importance of Plant Medicines to Life on Earth.* White River Junction, VT: Chelsea Green, 2002.

———. *Sacred Plant Medicine: The Wisdom in Native American Herbalism.* Rochester, VT: Bear and Company, 2006.

Burke, L. M. "Caffeine and Sports Performance." *Applied Physiology Nutrition and Metabolism* 33, 6 (December 2008): 1319–1334.

Burke, L. M., B. Kiens, and J. L. Ivy. "Carbohydrates and Fat for Training and Recovery." *Journal of Sports Science* 22, 1 (January 2004): 15–30.

Camus, A. *The Myth of Sisyphus.* New York: Random House, 1955.

Carson, R. *Silent Spring.* New York: Houghton Mifflin, 1962.

Casa, D. J. "Exercise in the Heat, II: Critical Concepts in Rehydration, Exertional Heat Illnesses, and Maximizing Athletic Performance." *Journal of Athletic Training* 34, 3 (1991): 253–262.

Cerqueira, M. T., M. M. Fry, and W. E. Connor. "The Food and Nutrient Intakes of the Tarahumara Indians of Mexico." *American Journal of Clinical Nutrition* 32, 4 (April 1979): 905–915.

Christensen, D. L., G. van Hall, and L. Hambraeus. "Food and Macronutrient Intake of Male Adolescent Kalenjin Runners in Kenya." *British Journal of Nutrition* 88 (2002): 711–717.

Christianson, A. "Ergogenics for Endurance Athletes." *Nutrition Science News,* March 2000. Available online at http://www.newhope.com/nutritionsciencenews/NSN_backs/Mar_00/athletes.cfm.

Clegg, D. O., et al. "Glucosamine, Chondroitin Sulfate, and the Two in Combination for Painful Knee Osteoarthritis." *New England Journal of Medicine* 354, 8 (2006): 795–808.

Coggan, A. R., and E. F. Coyle. "Carbohydrate Ingestion During Prolonged Exercise: Effects on Metabolism and Performance." *Exercise and Sport Sciences Reviews* (1991): 1–40.

Coleman, E. *The New Organic Grower: A Master's Manual of Tools and Techniques for the Home and Market Gardener.* White River Junction, VT: Chelsea Green, 1995.

Consumer Reports. "Are Organic Foods as Good as They're Grown?" Press release, December 15, 1997.

Cook, C. D. *Diet for a Dead Planet*. New York: New Press, 2004.

Cooper, A. *Bitter Harvest: A Chef's Perspective on the Hidden Dangers in the Foods We Eat and What You Can Do About It*. New York: Routledge, 2000.

Daniels, J. L., A. F. Olshan, and D. A. Savitz. "Pesticides and Childhood Cancers." *Environmental Health Perspectives* 105 (1997): 1068–1077.

Duty, S. M., N. P. Singh, M. J. Silva, D. B. Barr, J. W. Brock, L. Ryan, R. F. Herrick, D. C. Christiani, and R. Hauser. "The Relationship Between Environmental Exposures to Phthalates and DNA Damage in Human Sperm Using the Neutral Comet Assay." *Environmental Health Perspectives* 111, 9 (July 2003): 1164–1169.

Economos, C. D., S. S. Bortz, and M. E. Nelson. "Nutritional Practices of Elite Athletes: Practical Recommendations." *Sports Medicine* 16, 6 (1993): 381–399.

Ellis, C., and I. Cheney, directors. *King Corn: You Are What You Eat*. DVD. Mosaic Films, London, 2006.

Fallon, S., with M. G. Enig. *Nourishing Traditions: The Cookbook That Challenges Politically Correct Nutrition and the Diet Dictocrats*. Washington, DC: New Trends, 2001.

Ganio, M. S., J. F. Klau, D. J. Casa, L. E. Armstrong, and C. M. Maresh. "Effect of Caffeine on Sport-Specific Endurance Performance: A Systematic Review." *Journal of Strength and Conditioning Research* 23, 1 (2009): 315–324.

Garcia, D. K., director. *The Future of Food*. DVD. Lily Films, Mill Valley, CA, 2004.

"Glucosamine and Chondroitin—Topic Overview." http://www.webMd.

Grandjean, A. C. "Diets of Elite Athletes: Has the Discipline of Sports Nutrition Made an Impact?" *Journal of Nutrition* 127, 5 (Supplement, May 1997): 874S–877S.

Harris, B., D. Burress, and S. Eicher. *Demands for Local and Organic Produce: A Brief Review of the Literature*. Lawrence: Institute for Public Policy and Business Research, University of Kansas, 2000.

Hebbelinck, M. "Vegetarian Nutrition, Physical Activity, and Athletic Performance." *EVU News* 2 (1996), http://www.ivu.org/congress/euro95/athletic.html.

Horvath, P. J., C. K. Eagen, M. S. Stacie, D. Ryer-Calvin, and D. R. Pendergast. "The Effects of Varying Dietary Fat on the Nutrient Intake in Male and Female Runners." *Journal of the American College of Nutrition* 19, 1 (2000): 42–51.

Ivy, J. L. "Dietary Strategies to Promote Glycogen Synthesis After Exercise." *Canadian Journal of Applied Physiology* 26 (Supplement, 2001): S236–245.

Ivy, J. L., H. W. Goforth Jr., B. M. Damon, T. R. McCauley, E. C. Parsons, and T. B. Price. "Early Postexercise Muscle Glycogen Recovery Is Enhanced with a Carbohydrate-Protein Supplement." *Journal of Applied Physiology* 93, 4 (2002): 1337–1344.

Ivy, J. L., P. T. Res, R. C. Sprague, and M. O. Widzer. "Effect of a Carbohydrate-Protein Supplement on Endurance Performance During Exercise of Varying Intensity." *International Journal of Sport Nutrition and Exercise Metabolism* 13, 3 (2003): 382–395.

Jeavons, J. *How to Grow More Vegetables Than You Ever Thought Possible on Less Land Than You Can Imagine*. Berkeley, CA: Ten Speed Press, 1995.

Jones, G. "Caffeine and Other Sympathomimetic Stimulants: Modes of Action and Effects on Sports Performance. *Essays in Biochemistry* 44 (2008): 109–123.

Katz, S. E. *Wild Fermentation: The Flavor, Nutrition, and Craft of Live-Cultured Foods*. White River Junction, VT: Chelsea Green, 2003.

Keisler, B. D., and T. D. Armsey II. "Caffeine as an Ergogenic Aid." *Current Sports Medicine Reports* 5, 4 (June 2006): 215–219.

Kerksick, C., T. Harvey, J. Stout, B. Campbell, C. Wilborn, R. Kreider, D. Kalman, T. Ziegenfuss, H. Lopez, J. Landis, J. L. Ivy, and J. Antonio. "International Society of Sports Nutrition Position Stand: Nutrient Timing." *Journal of the International Society of Sports Nutrition* 5 (2008): 17.

Klein, S. "Lipid Metabolism During Exercise." Abstract from NIH Workshop: The Role of Dietary Supplements for Physically Active People. Health-World Online, http://www.healthy.net/scr/article.asp?ID=1672.

Maroon, J. C., and J. W. Bost. "N-3 Fatty Acids (Fish Oil) as an Anti-inflammatory: An Alternative to Nonsteroidal Anti-inflammatory Drugs for Discogenic Pain." *Surgical Neurology* 65 (2006): 326–331.

Matthys, D., P. Calders, J.-L. Pannier, and W. Derave. "Effect of Branched-Chain Amino Acids (BCAA), Glucose, and Glucose Plus BCAA on Endurance Performance in Rats." *Medicine and Science in Sports and Exercise* 3, 44 (1999): 583–587.

Maughan, R. J., and T. D. Noakes. "Fluid Replacement and Exercise Stress: A Brief Review of Studies on Fluid Replacement and Some Guidelines for the Athlete." *Sports Medicine* 12, 1 (1991): 16–31.

McArdle, W. D., F. I. Katch, and V. L. Katch. *Exercise Physiology, Energy, Nutrition, and Human Performance,* 3rd ed. Philadelphia: Lea and Febiger, 1991.

McCauley, L. A., et al. "Studying Health Outcomes in Farmworker Populations Exposed to Pesticides." *Environmental Health Perspectives* online, http://www.ehponline.org/members/2006/8526/8526.html.

Mero, A. "Leucine Supplementation and Intensive Training." *Sports Medicine* 27, 6 (1999): 347–358.

Midkiff, K. *The Meat You Eat: How Corporate Farming Has Endangered America's Food Supply.* New York: St. Martin's Press, 2004.

Miller, D. *The Jungle Effect: A Doctor Discovers the Healthiest Diets from Around the World—Why They Work and How to Bring Them Home.* New York: HarperCollins, 2008.

Miller, S. L., P. C. Gaine, C. M. Maresh, L. E. Armstrong, C. B. Ebbeling, L. S. Lamont, and N. R. Rodriguez. "The Effects of Nutritional Supplementation Throughout an Endurance Run on Leucine Kinetics During Recovery." *International Journal of Sports Nutrition and Exercise Metabolism* 17, 5 (2007): 456–467.

Mollison, B. *The Permaculture Book of Ferment and Human Nutrition.* Sisters Creek, Tasmania: Tagari Publications, 1993.

———. *Introduction to Permaculture.* Sisters Creek, Tasmania: Tagari Publications, 1997.

Moss, M., and A. Martin. "Food Problems Elude Private Inspectors." *New York Times,* March 5, 2009.

Nearing, S., and H. Nearing. *The Good Life.* New York: Schocken Books, 1990.

Nestle, M. *Safe Food.* Berkeley: University of California Press, 2003.

Organic Trade Association. "Measurable Effects of Pesticides on the Environment." http://www.ota.com/organic/health/environment/pesticides/environment.html.

———. "Organic Foods Production Act Backgrounder." http://www.ota.com/pp/legislation/backgrounder.html.

Paturel, A., and B. Wright. "Eat to Win: 4 Top Athletes Share Their Secrets to Healthy Eating." *Eating Well,* July 2008. Available online at http://www.eatingwell.com.

Pesticide Data Program. Annual Summary, Calendar Year 2005. Washington, DC: U.S. Department of Agriculture, 2006.

Price, W. A. *Nutrition and Physical Degeneration.* La Mesa, CA: Price-Pottenger Nutrition Foundation, 1939.

Rehrer, N. J. "Fluid and Electrolyte Balance in

Ultra-endurance Sport." *Sports Medicine* 31, 10 (2001): 701–715.

Robin, Monique-Marie, director. *The World According to Monsanto*. DVD. Arte Video, France, 2009.

Sampat, P. *Deep Trouble: The Hidden Threat of Groundwater Pollution*. Worldwatch Paper 154, December 2000.

Saunders, M. J., M. D. Kane, and M. K. Todd. "Effects of a Carbohydrate-Protein Beverage on Cycling Endurance and Muscle Damage." *Medicine and Science in Sports and Exercise* 36, 7 (July 2004): 1233–1238.

Savory, A. *Holistic Resource Management*. Washington, DC: Island Press, 1988.

Schmid, R. *Traditional Foods Are Your Best Medicine*. Rochester, VT: Healing Arts Press, 1997.

———. *The Untold Story of Milk: The History, Politics, and Science of Nature's Perfect Food—Raw Milk from Pasture-Fed Cows*. Washington, DC: New Trends, 2009.

Severson, K., and A. Martin. "It's Organic, but Does That Mean It's Safer?" *New York Times,* March 3, 2009.

Siahkohian, M., H. Farhadi, A. Naghizadeh Baghi, and A. Valizadeh. "Effect of Carbohydrate Ingestion on Sprint Performance Following Continuous Exercise." *Journal of Applied Sciences* 8, 4 (2008): 723–726.

Simopoulos, A. P. 1999. "Essential Fatty Acids in Health and Chronic Disease." *American Journal of Clinical Nutrition* 70, 3 (September 1999): 560–569.

Smith, J. M. *Seeds of Deception: Exposing Industry and Government Lies About the Safety of the Genetically Engineered Foods You're Eating*. Fairfield, IA: Yes! Books, 2003.

Snider, I. P., T. L. Bazzarre, and S. D. Murdoch. "Effects of Coenzyme Athletic Performance System as an Ergogenic Aid on Endurance Performance to Exhaustion." *International Journal of Sport Nutrition* 2 (1992): 272–286.

Soule, J., and J. K. Piper. *Farming in Nature's Image: An Ecological Approach to Agriculture*. Washington, DC: Island Press, 1991.

Strong, L. L., B. Thompson, G. D. Coronado, W. C. Griffith, E. M. Vigoren, and I. Islas. "Health Symptoms and Exposure to Organophosphate Pesticides in Farmworkers." *American Journal of Industrial Medicine* 46 (2004): 599–606.

True Food Network. http:// www.truefoodnow.org.

United States Department of Agriculture. Data and Statistics, http://www.usda.gov/wps/portal/!ut/p/_s.7_0_A/7_0_1OB?navid=DATA_STATISTICS.

———. National Agricultural Library. "Organic Food/Organic Production Information Access Tools." http://www.nal.usda.gov/afsic/pubs/ofp/ofp.shtml.

Von Duvillard, S. P., W. A. Braun, M. Markofski, R. Beneke, and R. Leithäuser. "Fluids and Hydration in Prolonged Endurance Performance." *Nutrition* 20, 7–8 (July–August 2004): 651–656.

Weston, S. B., S. Zhou, R. P. Weatherby, and S. J. Robson. "Does Exogenous Coenzyme Q10 Affect Aerobic Capacity in Endurance Athletes?" *International Journal of Sport Nutrition* 7 (1997): 197–206.

Williams, M. B., P. B. Raven, D. L. Fogt, and J. L. Ivy. "Effects of Recovery Beverages on Glycogen Restoration and Endurance Exercise Performance." *Journal of Strength and Conditioning Research* 17 (2003): 12–19.

Yates, A., J. Norwig, J. C. Maroon, J. Bost, J. P. Bradley, M. Duca, D. A. Wecht, R. Grove, A. Iso, I. Cobb, N. Ross, and M. Borden. "Evaluation of Lipid Profiles and the Use of Omega-3 Essential Fatty Acid in Professional Football Players." *Sports Health: A Multidisciplinary Approach* 1 (2009): 21.

Zuliani, U., A. Bonetti, and M. Campana. "The Influence of Ubiquinone (CoQ10) on the Metabolic Response to Work." *Journal of Sports Medicine and Physical Fitness* 29 (1989): 57–62.

Index

Hypoglycemia, 71
Hyponatremia, 82

Immune system, 19, 64, 66, 75, 87
Injuries, 12, 26, 32, 52, 59, 70, 78
Instant growth factor (IGF-1), 19
Instincts, following, 39–41
Insulin, 71, 73, 78, 79
Iron, 22, 66, 96, 182
Island Grilled Shrimp, 196–197
Island Rub, 196
Isoflavins, 182
Isoflavone, 112
Isoleucine, 69, 174
Ivy, John, 39–40, 72, 75

Jalapeño, salsa with, 142–143
Juices, 32, 41, 100; recipes for, 101–104
Jurek, Scott, 3

Kahl, Linda, 21
Kale, 29, 44, 233; chicken with, 224; duck with, 225; juice with, 103; steamed, 199
Kasha, 238; duck with, 225
Katch-McArdle formula, 53
Kimchi, 43, 145
Kitchen equipment, 257–258
Klein, Barbara, 28

Labels, 5, 7–8, 37–39, 47
Lamb, 27, 230–231
Leftovers, 43, 45, 49, 93
Legumes, 31, 65, 96
Lemon-Olive Oil Dressing, 117
Lemon Tahini Dressing, 130
Lentil Burgers, 128, 180–181
Lentils: burgers with, 180–181; salad with, 128
Leonard, Rodney, 6
Lettuce, 22, 27, 118–119
Leucine, 69, 174
Lifestyle, 10, 33, 43, 56, 60, 214; active, 2, 12–13, 36, 37, 50, 54, 61, 94; changes in, 32, 55; diet and, 30; exercise and, 11–12;

nutrition and, 3, 13, 23, 35–36, 47, 48, 59, 93
Lime: fish with, 200–201; juice with, 104
Linguine, 152–153
Linguine with Clams, Mint, and Tomatoes, 152–153
Local, buying/eating, 4–5, 30–31, 32, 96, 150

Macaroons, 73, 244
Macronutrients, 60, 61, 63–67, 78
Mad cow disease, 19
Magnesium, 22, 66, 82, 83, 96, 112
Maltodextrin, 7, 63
Maltose, 63
Mandoline, using, 123 (fig.)
Maple crème fraîche, 242–243
Maple Walnuts, 245
Marinated Beet Salad with Sugar Snap Peas and Cabbage Slaw, 122–123
Marinated Cucumber Salad, 168, 211
Maroon, Joseph, 10
Mayonnaise, 227; recipe for, 192
Meals: big/small, 42, 55–56; liquid, 86; post-training, 78–79; pre-training, 71; skipping, 55
Measurements, baking/cooking, 263
Meat, 27, 28, 31, 65, 70; buying, 3–4; growth/preparation of, 18, 19; recipes for, 230–236. See also Beef
Meatballs, soba noodles with, 166–167
Medium-chain triglycerides (MCTs), 55, 65, 107
Metabolism, 10, 13, 40, 41, 42, 49, 52, 54, 63, 71, 79, 103, 250; aerobic, 174; breakfast and, 55; cellular, 83
Micronutrients, 63–67, 78, 108, 112, 126
Milk, 19, 31, 79, 249
Minerals, 10, 11, 22, 28, 32, 49, 50, 66, 67, 108; live, 31; organic/

conventional crops compared, 22 (fig.)
Minestrone, 114
Mint: chicken with, 208–209; juice with, 102, 104; pasta with, 152–153
Miso, 43; dressing with, 131; soup with, 73, 112–113
Miso Soup, 73, 112–113
Mitchell, Jamie, 23, 93
Mollison, Bill, 145
Monkfish, recipe for, 204–205
Monoculture, 16, 20, 25, 29
Monsanto, Roundup and, 21
Morning Muffins, 250–251
Morning Quinoa, 252
Muffins, recipe for, 250–251
Muller, Nicolas, 93
Muscles, 73, 79, 80, 83; lean, 64–65; soreness, 12, 78, 145
Mushrooms, 30; chicken with, 208–209
Mustard, pork with, 236

National Organic Program (NOP), 23, 24
National Organic Standards Board (NOSB), 23
Nestle, Marion, 6, 17
Nonsteroidal antiinflammatory drugs (NSAIDs), 10
Noodles, 95; soba, 73, 164, 165–171, 199, 201, 211
Northeast Organic Farming Association (NOFA), 24
Nut butter, 41, 43, 45, 66, 73, 79, 250
Nutrients, 5, 9, 25–26, 37, 38, 42, 50, 55, 59, 73, 76, 95, 145; assimilating, 40, 71, 96; balance and, 45, 60, 62; breakdown of, 75; consumption of, 79; deficiency in, 49; diversity of, 72; enhancing, 97; exercise and, 81 (table); fat-soluble, 54; loss of, 22–23, 29, 38; preserving, 28, 29; required, 41, 60; seasonal, 8;

timing, 70, 75, 84; value, 4, 48; whole, 51, 60

Nutrition, 1–2, 5, 32, 33, 35, 42, 49, 51, 66; breaking point with, 41; choices with, 47, 59; focusing on, 53, 74; habits, 52; health issues and, 23; holistic approach to, 53; hydration and, 82; importance of, 92, 93, 94; increasing, 15; information, 12, 48; lifestyle and, 3, 13, 23, 36, 47, 48, 93; log, 82; performance and, 2–3, 23, 93; post-training, 77–79; pre-race, 86; pre-training, 70–73; problems with, 25, 42, 59; race-day, 74, 80, 86, 87, 88; recovery and, 60, 77, 166; required, 11, 56, 60; sports, 12, 13, 39, 50, 59, 60, 73; tactics for, 84; training and, 73–77

Nutrition plans, 2, 59, 69, 71, 77, 79, 87

Nuts, 41, 43, 72; dehydrating, 98; soaking/sprouting, 96–98, 98 (table), 259

Oatmeal, 63, 252
Ohno, Apollo Anton, 40
Oils, 258–259; coconut, 65; cooking, 95–96; dressings and, 116; palm, 65; partially hydrogenated, 37; polyunsaturated, 116
Omega-3 fatty acids, 9, 10, 27, 31, 62, 248
Omega-6 fatty acids, 9
Omega Hummus with Bee Pollen, 256
Oregon Tilth Association (OTA), 24
Organic, 9, 16, 32, 35, 48; buying, 3–4, 5; certification, 6, 23, 25; function/fashion of, 24; small farmers and, 25
Organic Foods Production Act (1990), 23
Organics: agribusiness vs., 16–20; choosing, 21–25
Orzo, 156–157

Oven-Roasted Chicken with Four Aromatic Variations, 214–219
Overeating, 40, 41, 42, 65, 66, 71, 85

Packaging, 5, 37–39, 49
Pan-Roasted Chicken, 221
Pan-Seared Red Snapper with Thai Citrus Sauce, 198–199
Pantry, essentials in, 45, 258–260
Papillote pouch, making, 190–191 (fig.)
Parsley: chicken with, 212–213; juice with, 103
Pasta, 38, 39, 63, 79, 95, 150–151, 233; chicken with, 220; recipes for, 152–157
Pasta with Fresh Roma Tomato Sauce and Meat (Turkey or Beef), Shrimp, or Scallops, 154–155
Pasteurization, 5, 6, 29
Peaches, 28, 44; recipe with, 242–243
Peanut butter, 253
Peanut sauce, 168, 169, 211
Pear, Kale, Parsley, and Celery Juice, 103
Pears, 45, 253; juice with, 103
Peas, 27, 29; chicken with, 208–209
Penne, 151, 152–153
Performance, 13, 48, 51, 70, 78, 84, 93; breakdown of, 80; caffeine and, 67; food and, 25, 33, 36; health and, 49; improving, 2–3, 7, 12, 32, 36, 49, 65, 69, 71; loss of, 26, 72; nutrition and, 2–3, 23, 93; supplements and, 50
Pesticides, 4, 7, 16, 17, 18, 20, 24
Phosphate, 82, 83
Phytic acid, 96, 145
Phytonutrients, 188
Pineapple, 28; juice with, 102
Pineapple, Cucumber, Ginger, and Mint Juice, 102
Polenta, 135, 158, 219, 233, 234, 235; recipes with, 159–163
Polenta Crab Cakes, 159

Polenta "Lasagna," 158, 162
Polenta with Egg, Goat Cheese, and Sprouts, 160
Popcorn, 43, 254–255
Pork, 37, 156, 171, 236; noodles with, 164; slow-roasted, 234–235
Pork chops, recipe for, 232–233
Porky Reuben with Kraut, Cheddar, and Mustard, 236
Portion control, 52, 73
Portman, Robert, 75
Potassium, 82, 83, 104
Potatoes, 30, 44, 63
Poultry, recipes for, 208–227
Power Granola, 248–249
Preparation, 35, 44, 45, 84, 93, 257; guidelines for, 95, 96; importance of, 42–43
Pribyl, Louis, 20
Price, Weston, 30–31, 32
Probiotics, 29, 50
Produce: buying, 3–4; organic, 28, 48
Proteins, 62, 65–66, 75, 108, 134, 174, 188; breakdown/assimilation of, 77, 145; carbohydrates and, 72, 76, 85; consumption of, 61, 76; creation of, 41; post-training, 79; soy, 66; storage of, 74; synthesis, 78

Quality: food, 3, 16, 21, 23, 37, 43, 44, 56, 57, 95; nutrient, 9, 72
Quinoa, 31, 44, 63, 65, 72, 174, 201, 204, 209, 238, 245; recipes for, 175–178, 252; salads and, 45
Quinoa Tabouleh, 178
Quinoa Veggie Burgers, 176–177

Raspberries, 37–38; smoothie with, 108
Raw Broccoli Soup, 111
Raw Sauerkraut, 68, 145–147
Raw Tomato Sauce, 163
Recovery, 1, 67, 69, 70, 71, 75, 79, 103; drinks, 66, 78; improving, 32; nutrition and, 60, 77, 166

About the Author

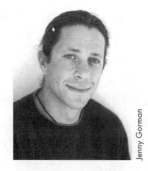

Jenny Gorman

Adam Kelinson is the face of Organic Performance, which grew out of his experience as an endurance athlete and professional chef, combined with his lifelong commitment to the environment.

As a private chef and nutritional consultant, Adam has cooked for many respected athletes, celebrities, and executives and has written on diet and nutrition for *TrailRunner, Inside Triathlon,* xtri.com, Dietwatch.com, and mariska.com. He has also served as nutritional director for the Silverman Full Distance Triathlon.

Adam graduated in 1996 from the University of Vermont with a degree in natural resources after designing his own major around sustainable agriculture and ecosystem management. Before beginning his career as a chef, he worked as an emergency medical technician and as a whitewater rafting and backcountry guide. An avid outdoorsman, he has passionately pursued the activities of rock and ice climbing, winter mountaineering, skiing, trail running, and more recently surfing.

Adam's love of cooking began in his mother's kitchen at the age of five. He attended Cook Street School of Fine Cooking in Denver, where he received Chef of Culinary Arts, Chef of Wine Arts, and Sommelier certifications in 2000. He has worked with some of the country's top chefs.

Adam has competed as a triathlete since 2000 and is a three-time Ironman finisher. He knows firsthand, as well as from years of study, that the right food can make a difference in performance, recovery, and rehabilitation

At Organic Performance, Adam and his team offer consulting and chef services to individuals and organizations, including sports teams. Organic Performance takes a pioneering approach that integrates traditional foods and ethnic cuisines into modern-day living and thinking. By demonstrating how everyone can use seasonally based, local, and organic foods as the foundation for success, Organic Performance's personalized services reconnect individuals to their bodies and the earth. For more information on Adam and his work, go to www.organicperformance.com.